Wound Healing - Mechanisms and Pharmacological Interventions

Edited by Guadalupe Tirma González-Mateo and Valeria Kopytina

Published in London, United Kingdom

Wound Healing - Mechanisms and Pharmacological Interventions
http://dx.doi.org/10.5772/intechopen.1008032
Edited by Guadalupe Tirma González-Mateo and Valeria Kopytina

Contributors
Alexandre Porcello, Alexis Laurent, Arzu Dinç Yavaş, Carolina Fonseca, Clarice Condeno, Cíntia Marques, Daniel Salas-Treviño, Daniel Santiago Cortés-Sarmiento, Diego Morales-Suarez, Eugenia Paris Coronado, Gabriel Ángel Mecott-Rivera, Guadalupe Tirma González-Mateo, Jens J. Rassweiler, Jorge Adrián Garza-Cerna, Jorge López Berroa, José Juan Pérez-Trujillo, Juan Manuel Herrera-Arbelaez, Juvido Agatep, Kelly Lourenço, Lee Ann Applegate, Mihaela Pertea, Nathalie Hirt-Burri, Pascual Bernal-Ovalle, Phumlane S. Mdluli, Roberto Montes de Oca-Luna, Tintswalo N. Mgwenya, Valeria Kopytina, Wolfgang Schaden, Xi Chen, Yanko Castro-Govea, Zhifeng Liao

First published in London, United Kingdom, 2025 by IntechOpen
IntechOpen is the global imprint of INTECHOPEN LIMITED, registered in England and Wales, registration number: 11086078, 167-169 Great Portland Street, London, W1W 5PF, United Kingdom

For EU product safety concerns: IN TECH d.o.o., Prolaz Marije Krucifikse Kozulić 3, 51000 Rijeka, Croatia, info@intechopen.com or visit our website at intechopen.com.

British Library Cataloguing-in-Publication Data
A catalogue record for this book is available from the British Library

Wound Healing - Mechanisms and Pharmacological Interventions
Edited by Guadalupe Tirma González-Mateo and Valeria Kopytina
p. cm.
Print ISBN 978-1-83634-764-4
Online ISBN 978-1-83634-763-7
eBook (PDF) ISBN 978-1-83634-765-1

Meet the editor

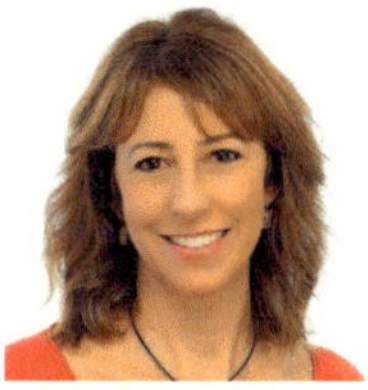

Guadalupe Tirma González-Mateo is a biomedical scientist specializing in translational research, preclinical models, molecular biology, and biostatistics. She currently oversees the scientific area at Premium Research SL, coordinating R&D initiatives in biomedical innovation and health technologies, including projects focused on regenerative medicine, bioinformatics, and AI-driven biomedical innovation. With a background that bridges molecular biology, inflammation, fibrosis, angiogenesis, cardiovascular disease, regenerative processes, and nephrology, she integrates preclinical and clinical insights, as well as data science, to accelerate the translation of laboratory findings into real-world applications. She has authored more than thirty scientific publications and holds a national award-winning patent. In academia, she lectures at the university level and has supervised undergraduate, master's, and doctoral theses, serving also on doctoral committees. She collaborates with hospitals, research centers, and technology companies to design multidisciplinary solutions for precision medicine and advanced therapies. Her work links academia and industry, focusing on mechanisms of tissue repair, biomaterials, wound healing, and the molecular pathways underlying chronic diseases.

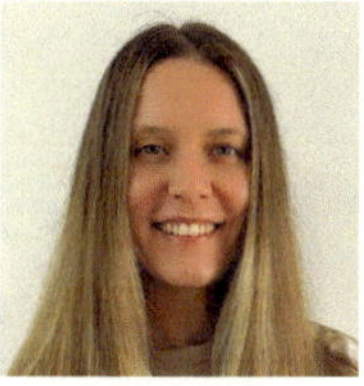

Valeria Kopytina holds a Ph.D. in Molecular Biosciences from the Autonomous University of Madrid and brings a multidisciplinary perspective to research management and clinical study coordination. With extensive experience in academic research and strategic project development, she leads the design and coordination of clinical studies. Dr. Kopytina has also contributed to multiple scientific publications, international conferences, and editorial boards, reflecting her commitment to advancing knowledge in the field.

Contents

Preface

Wound healing remains one of the most intricate and multifactorial processes in human biology. It is a dynamic and highly coordinated sequence of molecular, cellular, and systemic events aimed at restoring the integrity and function of damaged tissue. However, despite significant advances in biomedical science, chronic wounds continue to pose major global health challenges, impacting patients' quality of life and placing a considerable burden on healthcare systems.

Wound Healing – Mechanisms and Pharmacological Interventions brings together experts from diverse fields related to tissue repair to provide an integrative and translational overview of the science behind this process. The volume explores the biological mechanisms that regulate inflammation, angiogenesis, and extracellular matrix remodeling, while bridging them with clinical and pharmacological perspectives that inform real-world treatment.

The book follows a narrative path from molecular and biomarker discovery to objective clinical assessment, enzymatic and biophysical interventions, and regenerative strategies. It emphasizes the interplay between biological pathways and therapeutic innovation, reflecting how mechanistic understanding directly shapes pharmacological and clinical decision-making.

Recent years have initiated a paradigm shift in wound science, moving from the concept of "repair" toward true "regeneration", driven by advances in pharmacology and biotechnology. Looking ahead, data science and material innovation may further enhance therapeutic strategies in wound management. Artificial intelligence and machine learning have the potential to enable automated wound analysis and predictive modeling of healing trajectories. Bioinformatics and multi-omics approaches are likely to play a crucial role in uncovering new biomarkers and therapeutic targets. Nanotechnology and smart biomaterials are expected to improve drug delivery, modulate inflammation, and promote tissue integration. Together, these emerging directions may help shape a new era of precision wound medicine, where molecular insight, computational power, and regenerative technology converge.

Ultimately, this book aspires to provide readers with both scientific depth and clinically relevant information. By integrating molecular mechanisms, pharmacological interventions, and technological innovations, it provides a comprehensive understanding of how wounds heal and how they can be healed more effectively.

We hope that this volume will inspire clinicians, researchers, and students to continue advancing the science and art of wound healing, transforming traditional approaches into intelligent, regenerative, and patient-centered care for the years to come.

Guadalupe Tirma González-Mateo
Premium Research, S.L.,
Guadalajara, Spain

Valeria Kopytina
SEMERGEN, Spanish Society of Primary Care Physicians,
Madrid, Spain

Section 1

Biological and Molecular Insights

Chapter 1

Biomarkers in Wound Healing

Tintswalo N. Mgwenya and Phumlane S. Mdluli

Abstract

Biomarkers are transforming the study and management of wound healing by providing quantifiable indicators of tissue repair, prognosis, and therapeutic response. This chapter brings together existing insights on biomarkers associated with various stages of wound healing. It highlights progress in their detection and measurements and assesses their practical application in tracking progression, informing treatment decisions, and aiding drug development. This chapter emphasizes the integration of recent discoveries, showcasing how biomarker research is transforming wound healing from mere descriptive observation to predictive, precision-based methodologies.

Keywords: wound healing, biomarkers, detection, wound biomarkers, clinical application

1. Introduction

Wound healing is an intricate, dynamic, and highly regulated process involving various cellular and molecular events interactions that work together to restore tissue integrity after an injury [1]. This intricate process is divided into four orderly phases, namely hemostasis, inflammation, proliferative, and remodeling. Any disruption or delays in these phases can lead to impaired healing. This results in chronic wounds or excessive scarring, which pose considerable clinical and economic challenges worldwide [2]. Recently, there has been an increasing focus on discovering biomarkers that can offer insight into wound healing status, forecast outcome, and inform therapeutic interventions [3].

Biomarkers are generally characterized as quantifiable indicators for biological processes, disease states, and response to medical treatment [4]. In wound healing, biomarkers present opportunities to function as diagnostic tools, prognostic indicators, or predictors of therapeutic effectiveness [5]. The role of biomarkers goes further than simply indicating the biological condition of a wound. They offer significant potential in the stratification of patients, allowing clinicians to customize interventions to specific wound characteristics and systemic conditions [6]. Recent progress in molecular biology, proteomics, and metabolomics has greatly broadened the range of potential biomarkers in wound healing [7]. This includes inflammatory, growth factors, components of the extracellular matrix (ECM), matrix-degrading enzymes, and new genomic and proteomic signatures. Despite these advances, biomarker discoveries are still difficult to apply in clinical practice due to assay standardization, temporal viability, and patient factors like age, comorbidities, and nutritional status [8].

2. Key biomarkers in wound healing

Wound healing is governed by a precisely coordinated sequence of cellular and molecular processes, each defined by the temporal expression of certain biomolecules. Biomarkers linked to these events provide mechanistic healing understanding and diagnostic and prognostic significance. The primary biomarkers in each stage of wound healing are delineated below, emphasizing their biological functions and clinical significance.

2.1 Hemostasis stage biomarkers in wound healing

Important biomarkers of the hemostasis phase consist of platelet-derived growth factor (PDGF), thrombin, and fibrinogen/fibrin degradation products (FDPs) [9]. PDGF, released from activated platelets, promotes the recruitment and proliferation of fibroblast and smooth muscle cells. Wound healing fibroblast and fibrin activity are seen in **Figure 1**. Thrombin affects inflammation and angiogenesis *via* protease-activated receptors in addition to fibrin clot formation. Fibrinogen/FDPs indicate clot formation and breakdown, which may affect wound stability early on [10]. After the effective establishment of hemostasis and the release of first pro-healing mediators, the wound healing process advances to the inflammatory phase.

2.2 Inflammation phase biomarkers in wound healing

Following hemostasis, inflammatory mediators facilitate the recruitment of neutrophils, macrophages, and lymphocytes to the wound site. The inflammatory

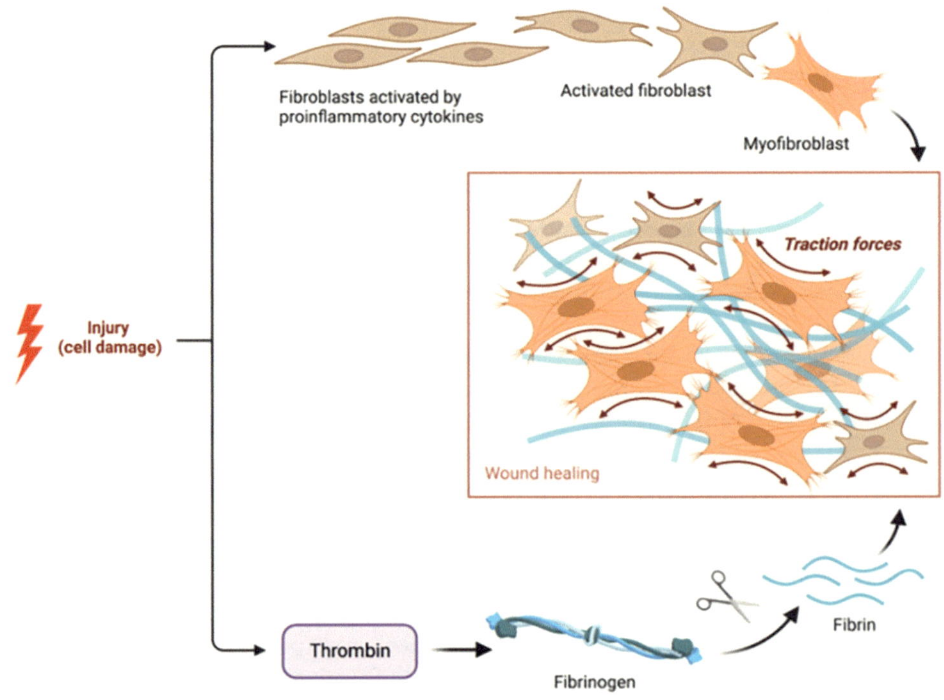

Figure 1.
Fibroblast and fibrin activity in wound healing. Fibroblasts migrate into the wound area, deposit ECM, and contract the tissue, while fibrin creates a temporary scaffold that stabilizes the clot and facilitates cell infiltration.

phase plays a crucial role in healing, aiding in the clearance of debris and pathogens from the wound area and preparing the groundwork for tissue repair [11]. Biomarkers associated with inflammation play a vital role in mediating and regulating these processes. Signaling proteins like cytokines and chemokines indicate inflammation. Interleukin-1β (IL-1β), interleukin-6 (IL-6), and tumor necrosis factor alpha (TNF-α) are the important biomarkers that govern the inflammatory response [12]. These pro-inflammatory cytokines play a crucial role in regulating leukocyte recruitment, activating endothelial cells, and modulating the acute phase response. C-reactive protein (CRP) is an acute-phase protein produced by the liver in response to IL-6 and functions as a systemic indicator of inflammation [13]. This protein also facilitates the control of the local inflammatory response by enhancing the recruitment and activation of immune cells.

High mobility group box 1 (HMGB1), a nuclear protein, serves as a danger-associated molecular pattern (DAMP) upon extracellular (EC) release, promoting inflammatory signaling [14]. Monocyte chemoattractant protein-1 (MCP-1) draws in monocytes that differentiate into macrophages, which are crucial for the removal of necrotic tissue [15]. Prostaglandins and leukotrienes, functioning as lipid mediators, play a crucial role in the inflammatory phase. Prostaglandins, produced by the action of cyclooxygenase enzymes, contribute to vasodilation and the increase of vascular permeability. Leukotrienes, generated *via* the lipoxygenase pathway, are involved in leukocyte chemotaxis, aiding the movement of immune cells to the injury site [16]. Matrix metalloproteinases (MMPs) are enzymes that degrade ECM components and facilitate the removal of damaged tissue. MMPs (MMP-2 and MMP-9) are involved in remodeling processes and help in the release of further growth factors that support the healing process. Their activity must be carefully controlled by the tissue inhibitor of metalloproteinases (TIMPs) to avoid excessive tissue damage [17].

Overproduction of reactive oxygen species (ROS) can damage tissue, yet controlled production is necessary for pathogen eradication and cellular communication. Neutrophils and macrophages produce ROS to eradicate pathogens and trigger additional immune response [18]. Antioxidants maintain equilibrium by reducing oxidative stress. Cellular part neutrophils are the first-wound responders, followed by monocytes/macrophages, which remove debris and secrete factors that switch the wound from inflammatory to proliferative.

2.3 Proliferation phase biomarkers in wound healing

The proliferation phase, which occurs between days 3 and 10 after injury, includes active tissue regeneration, angiogenesis, fibroblast proliferation, ECM deposition, and re-epithelialization [19]. Biomarkers indicate and impact these biological events, indicating wound healing progression and potential treatment targets. At this point, numerous biomarkers play a vital role in coordinating cellular functions that support tissue repair and regeneration. Growth factors are undoubtedly the most crucial indicators during the proliferative phase. Important biomarkers associated with proliferative phase include growth factors such as vascular endothelial growth factor (VEGF), epidermal growth factor (EGF), fibroblast growth factors (FGF-2), PDGF, transforming growth factor-β (TGF-β), cytokines (IL-6 and IL-10), cellular proliferation markers (Ki-67, α-SMA), ECM component and remodeling enzymes (collagen III, MMP-2, and MMP-9), and angiogenesis markers (CD31) [20, 21].

VEGF plays a vital role in the proliferation of endothelial cells and the formation of new capillaries. EGF signals cell proliferation and migration by attaching to the

EGF receptor (EGFR) on target cells, promoting tissue regeneration. FGF-2 promotes the proliferation of fibroblasts and stimulates collagen synthesis. PDGF attracts and stimulates fibroblasts, which play a crucial role in producing collagen and ECM components vital for structural repair. TGF-β governs ECM synthesis and immunological regulation. Types I and III are structural proteins suggestive of ECM remodeling. IL-6 and IL-10 are essential in facilitating communication between immune cells and cells responsible for tissue formation. They increase fibroblast and endothelial cell activity to reduce inflammation and promote proliferation.

Ki-67 and α-SMA are implicated in two aspects of tissue healing: cellular proliferation (Ki-67 + fibroblast/endothelial cells/keratinocytes) and mechanical contraction and ECM deposition (α-SMA + myofibroblast, wound tightening, and collagen deposition) [19]. Angiogenesis markers (CD31) reflect functional maturity and growth factor activity in neovascularization and reflect structural angiogenesis. Collagen and MMPs provide essential structural support and act as a framework for the formation of new tissue. Proteoglycans and glycosaminoglycans, essential components of the ECM, are crucial for enabling cell signaling and establishing a hydrated environment that supports cell proliferation and migration.

2.4 Remodeling stage biomarkers in wound healing

The remodeling or maturation phase is the concluding and longest stage of wound healing. It starts 21 days after injury and can persist for months or years, depending on the wound and patient. This phase involves ECM maturation, collagen cross-linking, and a decrease in cellularity. Key biomarkers include tissue inhibitors of metalloproteinases (TIMPs), hydroxyproline, and lysyl oxidase (LOX) [21].

Collagen type I, a primary structural protein that replaces type III collagen, enhances wound tensile strength. Meanwhile, collagen type III, an early form of collagen, undergoes gradual degradation, indicating the transition into the remodeling phase [22]. MMP-1, MMP-2, MMP-9, and MMP-13 degrade ECM components for appropriate ECM remodeling. TIMP-1 and TIMP-2 regulate MMP activity to avert excessive ECM breakdown.

TGF-β1 facilitates the differentiation of fibroblast into myofibroblasts, enhances ECM production, and contributes to scar formation. α-SMA is a hallmark of myofibroblasts that facilitate wound contraction and matrix remodeling. Fibronectin is an ECM glycoprotein that plays a crucial role in matrix construction and cellular adhesion throughout the remodeling process. Decorin modulates collagen fibrillogenesis and TGF-β activity. LOX crosslinks collagen and elastin fibers, enhancing matrix stability and tensile strength. VEGF decreases during the remodeling phase; however, some wounds may still exhibit residual angiogenic activity.

During the remodeling stage, biomarkers include collagen I, MMPs, TIMPs, and TGF-β1 demonstrating inflammation resolution, balanced matrix remodeling, and tissue integrity restoration [19]. However, disruptions in these processes can result in impaired healing. When the biomolecular milieu of normal wound repair is disrupted by extended inflammation, increased protease activity, and inadequate growth factor signaling, the wound may become chronic [23]. **Table 1** summarizes the key biomarkers of each phase of wound healing. Understanding the biomarker profile change from normal remodeling to chronic wounds is crucial for identifying pathological processes and developing targeted therapies to enhance healing.

Phase	Key biomarkers	Role/function	Reference
Hemostasis	PDGF, thrombin Fibrinogen/fibrin	Initiate clot formation, platelet aggregation, and provision of matrix formation	[9, 10]
Inflammation	IL-1, TNF-α, IL-6, CRP, MPO	Pro-inflammatory cytokines and enzymes that recruit immune cells, clear debris, and prevent infection	[12–15]
Proliferation	VEGF, FGF, TGF-β, KGF, collagen type III	Stimulate angiogenesis, fibroblast proliferation, ECM deposition, and re-epithelialization	[19, 20]
Remodeling	MMPs (MMP-1, MMP-9), TIMPs, collagen type I, TGF-β (persistent)	ECM remodeling, collagen maturation, regulation of protease activity, and scar formation	[19–23]

Table 1.
Wound healing and key biomarkers.

3. Chronic wounds biomarkers

Inflammation, poor angiogenesis, and increased proteolytic activity persist in chronic wounds such as pressure ulcers, diabetic foot ulcers, and venous leg ulcers. Chronically elevated levels of IL-1β, TNF-α, and IL-6 indicate persistent inflammation [19]. Decreased VEGF and PDGF levels lead to compromised angiogenesis and impaired cellular migration, while elevated bacterial DNA and endotoxin levels are indicative of biofilm presence and underlying infection [24]. The continuous presence of these mediators hinders tissue regeneration, exacerbates tissue damage, prolongs inflammation, and obstructs advancement to the proliferative phase. Chronic wounds, accompanied by persistent inflammation, exhibit compromised angiogenesis, and altered ECM remodeling. Insufficient blood vessel formation due to low VEGF and other angiogenic factors prevents tissue regeneration by preventing oxygen and nutrition delivery [19].

At the same time, chronic wounds show increased levels of proteolytic enzymes, especially MMPs, which break down structural proteins and growth factors within the ECM. The heightened proteolytic activity compromises tissue integrity and hinders the cellular migration and proliferation necessary for effective wound healing. These pathological features create a poor wound environment, hindering healing and increasing the risk of infection, chronic pain, and amputation [24]. Angiogenesis is an essential component of the development of new blood vessels, enabling the reestablishment of oxygen and nutrient supply to repair tissue. PDGF and VEGF are critical pro-angiogenetic factors that aid in the stabilization of newly formed vessels and the proliferation and migration of endothelial cells. In chronic wounds or certain clinical situations, low PLDGF and VEGF levels directly inhibit the angiogenic process, limiting wound bed vascularization and tissue repair [25].

In addition to angiogenesis, these growth factors play a vital role in cellular migration, especially for fibroblasts and keratinocytes. Fibroblasts generate components of the ECM and collagen, while keratinocytes contribute to re-epithelialization. A potent fibroblast chemoattractant, PDGF plays a critical role in cell proliferation and migration, whereas VEGF primarily indicates angiogenesis by promoting endothelial cell proliferation and new vessel formation. The compromised regeneration environment is further intensified by persistent wounds or infected tissue, which often harbors high concentrations of bacterial DNA and endotoxins. Endotoxins, especially gram-negative bacteria's lipopolysaccharides (LPS), stimulate host immunological responses *via* toll-like receptors (TLRs) [26]. An elevated bacterial DNA load, usually detected *via* molecular assay, indicates ongoing bacterial colonization or infection. Biofilms develop a structured, self-protective matrix that makes bacteria resistant to immune clearance and antimicrobial therapies, resulting in a persistent infection source.

Biofilms worsen the detrimental wound environment by continuously generating planktonic bacteria, endotoxins, and diverse virulence factors that sustain local inflammation [27]. The presence of microbial products may exacerbate tissue injury, impede wound healing, and trigger pro-inflammatory cytokines such as IL-1β, TNF-α, and IL-6. The prolonged inflammatory environment hinders growth factor production and reparative cell recruitment and efficacy, sustaining chronic wounds [19].

Moreover, endotoxins found in the biofilm microenvironment can directly suppress the expression of PDGF and VEGF, worsening the issue of impaired angiogenesis. Studies show that bacterial components and persistent inflammation can impede the growth and movement of endothelial cells, leading to insufficient development of the vascular network [19, 28]. Reduced angiogenesis, impaired fibroblast migration, and continuing microbial stimulation cause hypoxia, necrosis, and exudate in non-healing wounds. A significant result of infections linked to biofilms is the disturbance of the ECM remodeling process [29]. Biofilms and their related endotoxins lead to elevated levels of MMPs while concurrently reducing TIMPs, causing unregulated degradation of the ECM. This undermines the framework crucial for cell migration and angiogenesis, thereby hindering the healing process. Without a strong ECM framework, endothelial cells and fibroblasts cannot migrate or multiply efficiently, resulting in persistent tissue damage [30].

In wounds affected by biofilm and lacking growth factors, therapeutic strategies present significant challenges. Conventional antibiotics struggle to penetrate biofilm matrices, and reduced pro-angiogenic signaling lowers the efficacy of growth factor-based treatments [31]. This emphasizes the need to combine antibacterial biofilm-disrupting agents with pro-angiogenic or ECM-stabilizing treatments to revitalize regenerative wounds. Lower PDGF and VEGF levels, along with higher bacterial DNA and endotoxin, indicate a severely impaired wound healing environment with disturbed angiogenesis, inadequate cellular migration, and biofilm-related infection [32]. Addressing these interconnected pathological features requires a complex, multifaceted therapeutic approach aimed at restoring vascularization, managing inflammation, and eliminating biofilms to ultimately promote effective tissue regeneration.

4. Clinical application of wound healing biomarkers

The importance of biomarkers in clinical setting is considerable, as they serve as key diagnostic indicators. Specific biomarkers can differentiate between acute and chronic wounds by highlighting the unique cellular and molecular activities associated with each type. Therapeutic monitoring involves evaluating therapy efficacy such as alterations in MMP levels subsequent to debridement. Non-healing wounds are frequently associated with elevated concentrations of pro-inflammatory cytokines and proteases such as MMPs, whereas their expeditious resolution is indicative of acute wound healing [33]. Doctors can tailor treatment to patients' biological wounds using this differentiation. Prognostic biomarkers complement diagnosis. By observing specific markers and their levels over time, healthcare professionals can predict healing outcomes and identify patients who might be at risk for insufficient recovery. Persistently high levels of inflammatory mediators or reduced concentrations of growth factors (e.g., VEGF) could indicate a compromised healing process [19]. Identifying at-risk patients early allows for prompt and focused interventions, improving outcomes and reducing the likelihood of complications.

Therapeutic monitoring constitutes a crucial application of biomarkers. Clinicians can assess a wound's reaction to specific treatments by observing changes in biomarker levels before and after the intervention. An illustration of this is the evaluation of MMP levels following debridement. A decrease in MMP levels following debridement indicates a better healing environment, while persistently elevated levels may signal tissue deterioration and the need for further treatment changes [34]. Infection surveillance entails the prompt identification of microbial colonization or biofilm development. Examples encompass point-of-care (POC) assessments for protease activity in the management of chronic wounds. Assessment of serum CPR and procalcitonin levels guide antibiotic treatment in instances of infected wounds [35]. Effective wound management necessitates the early identification of microbial colonization or biofilm formation by antibiotic-resistant bacteria. Increased levels of biomarkers such as IL-6 may signal the initial onset of infection, enabling prompt clinical action before clear signs and symptoms develop [36]. This proactive approach can help prevent complications such as sepsis or worsening of wounds associated with chronic infections.

The incorporation of biomarkers into regular wound care enhances personalized treatment. The specific needs of a patient's wound can be addressed by doctors through customized treatment approaches to account for the unique biological obstacles that are present. A wound showing elevated protease activity could benefit from protease-modulating dressings, while one lacking sufficient angiogenic activity may require interventions focused on enhancing blood vessel formation [37]. This method, informed by biomarkers, enhances treatment precision and boosts the likelihood of attaining favorable outcomes. Moreover, biomarkers are crucial in clinical research and the development of innovative therapies. Biomarkers serve as surrogate endpoints in clinical studies, providing objective and measurable assessments of the biological response to experimental therapies. This accelerates the evaluation of new wound care products and techniques, ultimately providing innovative solutions to patients more effectively. Innovative biomarker research is uncovering new wound biology, enabling the opportunity to improve existing treatments and discover new therapeutic targets.

The growing availability of POC biomarker tests holds promises for improving the feasibility of biomarker-driven wound management in everyday clinical settings. Portable devices and rapid tests that identify specific biomarker levels at the bedside facilitate real-time decision-making, enabling doctors to promptly modify therapies based on immediate feedback. This innovation improves wound care efficiency and efficacy in outpatient, home care, and resource-limited settings. In many non-healing wounds, elevated levels of proteases, especially MMPs, can degrade essential ECM components and growth factors, thereby impeding the healing process [38]. POC diagnostics allow clinicians to quickly assess protease activity at bedside, providing rapid insights into the biochemical environment of the wound [39]. Upon identification of elevated protease activity, targeted interventions, such as protease-modulating dressings or enhanced debridement, may be promptly implemented. This prompt enables the personalization of wound management, reducing the danger of prolonged inflammation and increasing the likelihood of tissue regeneration.

These markers help doctors identify localized inflammation from systemic infection and determine if antibiotics are needed [40]. This approach encourages responsible use of antimicrobials by reducing unnecessary antibiotic prescriptions and decreasing the risk of resistance. Furthermore, monitoring CPR and procalcitonin levels over time may reveal the patient's therapeutic response, allowing treatment plans to be adjusted based on objective, real-time biological data [41].

4.1 Introduction to emerging biomarkers and technologies in wound healing

Traditional biomarkers, such as cytokines, growth factors, and MMPs, have been thoroughly examined to assess wound development. The advent of improved molecular biology and high-throughput omics technology enables researchers to develop novel biomarkers that have enhanced sensitivity and specificity [42]. The new biomarkers improve comprehension of the molecular pathways in wound repair, offering prospects for breakthroughs in diagnostic, prognostic, and therapeutic techniques. MicroRNAs (miRNAs) are a category of small non-coding RNAs that regulate gene expression after transcription, and they are among the most significant discoveries. miRNA binds to complementary regions in messenger RNAs, leading to mRNA destruction or translation inhibition [43, 44]. Their involvement in numerous physiological and pathological processes has positioned them as crucial regulators in the wound healing process. Various miRNAs are linked to distinct phases of wound healing, affecting processes such as cell proliferation, inflammation, angiogenesis, and remodeling of the ECM. **Table 2** provides an overview of emerging biomarkers in wound healing.

miR-21 is one of the most thoroughly studied miRNAs regarding wound healing. This chemical has shown the capacity to promote angiogenesis. By concentrating on and suppressing anti-angiogenic factors such as phosphate and tensin homolog (PTEN), miR-21 enhances the migration of endothelial cells and the development of capillary tubes [49]. Elevated levels of miR-21 in wound tissue correlate with improved neovascularization, suggesting its possible therapeutic function in promoting healing, especially in ischemic or chronic wounds [49]. Conversely, miR-29 plays a vital role in the regulation of fibrosis, an essential process in wound healing and remodeling [50]. This miRNA targets and inhibits the expression of various ECM components, including several collagens. The reduced expression of miR-29 has been

Type of biomarker	Illustrative biomarker	Essential functions in wound healing	Reference
MicroRNAs	miR-21, miR-29	Modulate angiogenesis, fibrosis, and inflammation	[43–45]
Exosomes	MSC-derived exosomes, Kera-exosomes	Regulate inflammation, stimulate angiogenesis	[46]
Metabolites	Lactate, amino acids, lipids	Exhibit tissue metabolism, hypoxia, and healing	[47]
Proteins	VEGF, TGF-β, MMP-9	Demonstrate chronicity, fibrosis, and angiogenesis	[48]

Table 2.
Overview of emerging biomarkers and their roles.

associated with heightened matrix deposition and fibrotic conditions. Modulating miR-29 may facilitate the equilibrium of matrix production and degradation throughout the wound remodeling process, potentially preventing pathological scarring or the continuation of chronic wounds [50]. **Figure 2** depicts the regulatory mechanism of miR-21 and miR-29 in the process of wound healing.

4.2 Exosomes and EC vesicles: Innate mediators of cellular interaction

Exosomes and other EC vesicles (EVs) play a crucial role in facilitating cell-to-cell communication within the wound microenvironment [51]. **Table 3** summarizes exosome-based wound diagnosis and therapy. Diverse cell types release these nanoscale vesicles, which transport a payload of proteins, lipids, and nucleic acids, including miRNAs. Exosomes derived from mesenchymal stem cells, keratinocytes, and immune cells are crucial in the wound healing process as they modulate inflammation, promote angiogenesis, and enhance tissue regeneration [57]. The diagnostic potential of exosomes is rooted in their capacity to mirror the molecular condition of the cells from which they originate. Exosomal content can show biomarkers that indicate wound disease, including acute, chronic, and healing, providing a non-invasive diagnostic approach. For therapeutic purposes, exosomes can be produced or extracted from specific cell types to deliver regenerative signals directly to the wound sites. Studies show that therapies using exosomes accelerate wound healing, reduce inflammation, and improve outcomes in tissue regeneration [57, 58].

4.3 Metabolic profiling: Mapping biochemical alterations in wounds

Metabolomics, involving the comprehensive analysis of small-molecule metabolites within biological systems [59], has attracted attention in the field of wound

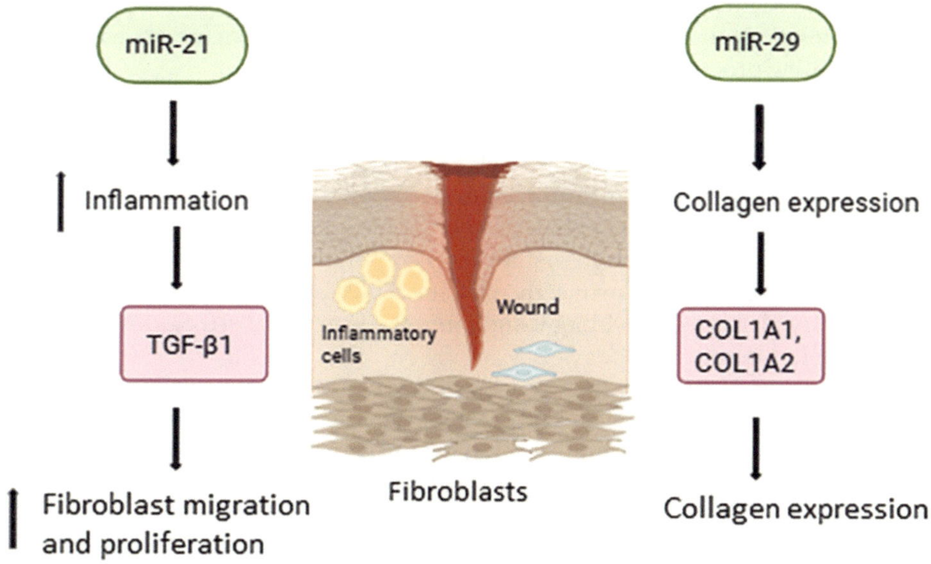

Figure 2.
The regulatory mechanism of miR-21 and miR-29 in the process of wound healing. The diagram demonstrates the role of miR-21 in promoting angiogenesis. Conversely, miR-29 suppresses the deposition of the ECM by downregulating collagen gene expression in fibroblasts, thus influencing fibrosis and ECM remodeling.

Exosome source	Diagnostic function	Therapeutic function	Reference
Mesenchymal stem cell-derived exosomes	Analyze cargo (miRNAs, proteins) to reflect inflammatory or regenerative wound microenvironments	Facilitates angiogenesis, decreases inflammation, increases fibroblasts, keratinocyte proliferation	[52]
Keratinocyte-derived exosomes	Assess epithelial cells status and re-epithelialization advancement of *via* molecular composition	Enhance migration and proliferation of keratinocytes, facilitating better wound closure	[53]
Endothelial cell-derived exosomes	Evaluate endothelial-specific biomarkers to evaluate angiogenic activity and vascular remodeling	Stimulate the formation of new blood vessels, aiding in tissue perfusion and repair	[54]
Immune cell-derived exosomes (e.g., microphages)	Assess the polarization of immune responses (M1 vs. M2 phenotypes) in wounds	Modulate inflammatory responses to encourage a shift from pro-inflammatory to regenerative phenotypes	[55]
Fibroblast-derived exosomes	Reflect ECM remodeling processes and signaling associated with fibrosis	Improve the deposition of the ECM, increase collagen production, and strengthen wound tensile strength	[56]

Table 3.
Exosome-based wound diagnosis and therapy. Exosomes from different cell types can be used as diagnostic biomarkers for wound status and therapeutically to improve tissue regeneration and modulate inflammatory responses.

research. Wound exudates consist of a variety of metabolites that reflect local metabolic processes [60]. **Figure 3** shows a procedure for metabolomic analysis of wound exudates. By profiling these metabolites, researchers can identify alterations in metabolic pathways occurring at different stages of wound healing or chronic, non-healing wounds. Alterations in amino acid, lipid, and energy metabolism have been linked to impaired healing processes [61].

Identifying unique metabolomic signatures associated with healing or chronic conditions offers valuable clinical insights. Specific metabolites, such as increased lactate or altered amino acid ratios, may signify continued inflammation or hypoxia in the wound [62]. Metabolic profiling helps us understand wound biochemistry and anticipate healing outcomes, allowing us to tailor treatment to the wound's metabolic state. To develop a more thorough system-level comprehension, it is important to analyze upstream regulators, primarily proteins. Thus, proteomics functions as a supplementary platform, providing insight into the functional effectors that influence these metabolic alterations.

Wound healing entails dynamic, stage-specific changes in metabolic and proteomic patterns. Metabolomics measures biological activity, while proteomics reveals protein expression, alteration, and location that affects these processes, providing a more complete mechanistic insight [63].

4.4 Proteomics analysis in wound research

Genomic and metabolomic research is enhanced by proteomics, which reveals dynamic changes in protein expression, alterations, and interactions in injured tissues [64]. A summary of protein biomarkers found from proteomic analysis of wound

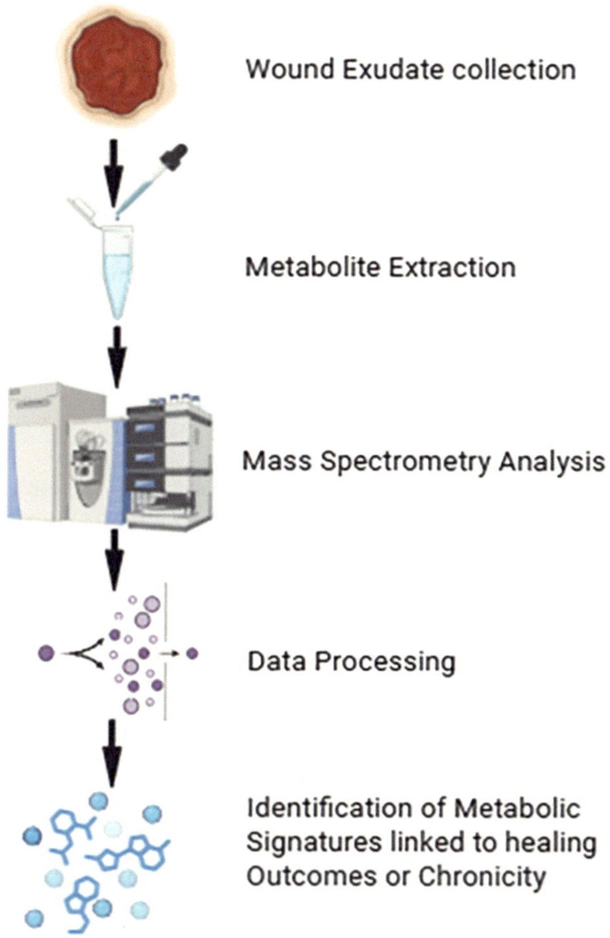

Figure 3.
Procedure for metabolomic analysis of wound exudates. The diagram illustrates the sequential steps involved in metabolic analysis, encompassing wound exudate collection, metabolite extraction, mass spectrometry, data processing, and the identification of metabolic signatures linked to healing outcomes or chronicity.

tissue and exudates is provided in **Table 4**. Wound exudates, tissue, and cellular secretomes serve as ample sources for proteomic analysis. Advanced mass spectrometry and bioinformatics can identify protein signatures that indicate chronic wound problems or healing stages. Proteomic analysis has uncovered a range of proteins whose expression levels correlate with effective healing or persistent inflammation. For instance, active tissue regeneration is linked to high amounts of fibronectin, VEGF, and TGF-β, while chronic wounds are linked to higher MMP-9 and inflammatory mediators [70]. Understanding these protein patterns can help clinicians evaluate wound health and identify appropriate treatments.

Metabolic profiling and proteomic analysis have become significant methods in enhancing our understanding of the intricate biochemical environment present in both healing and non-healing wounds. Metabolic profiling provides vital information about the wound environment and systemic factors that affect repair by mapping metabolic pathways such amino acids, energy, and oxidative stress [71]. In addition, proteomics helps uncover mediators and therapeutic targets by characterizing

Protein	Functional role in wound healing	Connection to healing or chronicity	Reference
VEGF	Encourages the formation of new blood vessels and the growth of endothelial cells	Increased in actively healing wounds; reduced in chronic or ischemic wounds	[65]
TGF-β	Promotes fibroblast activation, ECM deposition, and scar formation	Increased in both standard healing and fibrotic, hypertrophic scar tissue	[66]
MMP-9	Breaks down ECM components and regulates remodeling	Significantly increased in chronic, non-healing wounds leading to ECM degradation	[67]
Fibronectin	Facilitates cell adhesion, migration, and matrix organization	Increased during the initial and proliferative stages of acute wound healing	[9, 10]
IL-6	Mediates inflammatory response and the recruitment of immune cells	Increased during acute inflammation, consistently elevated in chronic wounds	[68]
Collagen I and III	Provides structural foundation for tissue repair and scar formation	Impaired healing or excessive fibrosis results from dysregulated deposition	[22]
S100A8/A9 (Calprotectin)	Regulates inflammation and supports antimicrobial defense	Heightened levels in chronic wounds, indicating ongoing inflammation	[69]

Table 4.
Overview of protein biomarkers found from proteomic analysis of wound tissue and exudates.

proteins involved in inflammation, angiogenesis, ECM remodeling, and immune control. Collectively, these high-throughput, systems-oriented methods are transforming wound research by identifying novel biomarkers, developing tailored therapy regimens, and improving clinical outcomes in acute and chronic wound management.

5. Conclusion

Biomarkers are essential in regulating and monitoring the intricate, interconnected stages of wound healing, starting with inflammatory markers such as IL-6, TNF-α, and neutrophil elastase during the hemostasis and inflammation phases, progressing to growth factors like VEGF and PDGF in the proliferation stage, and including ECM-related proteins such as collagen I, MMPs, and TGF-B1 in the remodeling phase. In chronic wounds, the ongoing elevation of inflammatory cytokines, the imbalance of MMP/TIMP ratios, and the disruption of growth factor signaling interfere with the normal healing process, leading to delayed recovery. The clinical application of wound healing biomarkers facilitates the development of personalized treatment strategies, enabling the targeted therapies that specifically address deficiencies or excesses within the healing cascade. Metabolic profiling and proteomics provide thorough investigations of wound management, revealing biomarkers and therapeutic targets. Recognizing and focusing on phase-specific and chronic wound biomarkers presents significant opportunities for improvements in prognosis, diagnosis, and treatment within the realm of wound care.

DOI: http://dx.doi.org/10.5772/intechopen.1012961

Acknowledgements

Tintswalo N. Mgwenya contributed substantially to the conception or design of the work and in drafting or revising the work; and Phumlane S. Mdluli revised the manuscript version to be published.

Conflict of interest

The authors declare no conflict of interest.

Author details

Tintswalo N. Mgwenya[1,2]* and Phumlane S. Mdluli[1]

1 Health Platform, Advanced Materials Division, Mintek, Randburg, Gauteng, South Africa

2 DSI/Mintek Nanotechnology Innovation Centre, Advanced Materials Division, Mintek, Randburg, Gauteng, South Africa

*Address all correspondence to: tintswalom@mintek.co.za

References

[1] Wallace HA, Basehore BM, Zito PM. Wound Healing Phases. Treasure Island (FL): StatPearls publishing; 2025. Available from: https://www.ncbi.nlm.nih.gov/books/NBK470443/

[2] Ozgok Kangal MK, Regan JP. Wound Healing. Treasure Island (FL): StatPearls Publishing; 2025. Available from: https://www.ncbi.nlm.nih.gov/books/NBK535406/

[3] Lu SH, Samandari M, Li C. Multimodal sensing and therapeutic systems for wound healing and management: A review. Sensors and Actuators Reports. 2022;**100075**:2666-0539

[4] Califf RM. Biomarker definitions and their applications. Experimental Biology and Medicine (Maywood, N.J.). 2018;**243**(3):213-221. DOI: 10.1177/1535370217750088

[5] Méndez Hernández R, Ramasco RF. Biomarkers as prognostic predictors and therapeutic guide in critically ill patients: Clinical evidence. Journal of Personalized Medicine. 2023;**13**(2):333. DOI: 10.3390/jpm13020333

[6] Weigelt MA, Lev-Tov HA, Tomic-Canic M, Lee WD, Williams R, Strasfeld D, et al. Advanced wound diagnostics: Toward transforming wound care into precision medicine. Advances in wound care (New Rochelle). 2022;**11**(6):330-359. DOI: 10.1089/wound.2020.1319

[7] Bai H, Arnedo AS, Liu Y, et al. Unraveling the molecular dynamics of wound healing: Integrating spatially resolved lipidomics and temporally resolved proteomics. Analytical and Bioanalytical Chemistry. 2025;**417**. DOI: 10.1007/s00216-025-05865-5

[8] Ou FS, Michiels S, Shyr Y, Adjei AA, Oberg AL. Biomarker discovery and validation: Statistical considerations. Journal of Thoracic Oncology. 2021;**16**(4):537-545. DOI: 10.1016/j.jtho.2021.01.1616

[9] Periayah MH, Halim AS, Mat Saad AZ. Mechanism action of platelets and crucial blood coagulation pathways in hemostasis. International Journal of Hematology-Oncology and Stem Cell Research. 2017;**11**(4):319-327

[10] Shlobin NA, Har-Even M, Itsekson-Hayosh Z, Harnof S, Pick CG. Role of thrombin in central nervous system injury and disease. Biomolecules. 2021;**11**(4):562. DOI: 10.3390/biom11040562

[11] Ellis S, Lin EJ, Tartar D. Immunology of wound healing. Current Dermatology Reports. 2018;7:350-358. DOI: 10.1007/s13671-018-0234-9

[12] Chen L, Deng H, Cui H, Fang J, Zuo Z, Deng J, et al. Inflammatory responses and inflammation-associated diseases in organs. Oncotarget. 2017;**9**(6):7204-7218. DOI: 10.18632/oncotarget.23208

[13] Singh B, Goyal A, Patel BC. C-Reactive Protein: Clinical Relevance and Interpretation. In: StatPearls [Internet]. Treasure Island (FL): StatPearls Publishing; 2025. Available from: https://www.ncbi.nlm.nih.gov/books/NBK441843/

[14] Agalave NM, Svensson CI. Extracellular high-mobility group box 1 protein (HMGB1) as a mediator of persistent pain. Molecular Medicine. 2015;**20**(1):569-578. DOI: 10.2119/molmed.2014.00176

[15] Deshmane SL, Kremlev S, Amini S, Sawaya BE. Monocyte chemoattractant protein-1 (MCP-1): An overview. Journal of Interferon & Cytokine Research. 2009;**29**(6):313-326. DOI: 10.1089/jir.2008.0027

[16] Ricciotti E, FitzGerald GA. Prostaglandins and inflammation. Arteriosclerosis, Thrombosis, and Vascular Biology. 2011;**31**(5):986-1000. DOI: 10.1161/ATVBAHA.110.207449

[17] Cabral-Pacheco GA, Garza-Veloz I, Castruita-De la Rosa C, Ramirez-Acuña JM, Perez-Romero BA, Guerrero-Rodriguez JF, et al. The roles of matrix metalloproteinases and their inhibitors in human diseases. International Journal of Molecular Sciences. 2020;**21**(24):9739. DOI: 10.3390/ijms21249739

[18] Bardaweel SK, Gul M, Alzweiri M, Ishaqat A, ALSalamat HA, Bashatwah RM. Reactive oxygen species: The dual role in physiological and pathological conditions of the human body. Eurasian Journal of Medicine. 2018;**50**(3):193-201. DOI: 10.5152/eurasianjmed.2018.17397

[19] Schultz GS, Chin GA, Moldawer L, et al. Principles of wound healing. In: Fitridge R, Thompson M, editors. Mechanisms of Vascular Disease: A Reference Book for Vascular Specialists. Adelaide (AU): University of Adelaide Press; 2011. p. 23. Available from: https://www.ncbi.nlm.nih.gov/books/NBK534261/

[20] Barrientos S, Stojadinovic O, Golinko MS, Brem H, Tomic-Canic M. Growth factors and cytokines in wound healing. Wound Repair and Regeneration. 2008;**16**(5):585-601. DOI: 10.1111/j.1524-475X.2008.00410.x

[21] Cai L, Xiong X, Kong X, Xie J. The role of the lysyl oxidases in tissue repair and remodeling: A concise review. Tissue Engineering and Regenerative Medicine. 2017;**14**(1):15-30. DOI: 10.1007/s13770-016-0007-0

[22] Singh D, Rai V, Agrawal DK. Regulation of collagen I and collagen III in tissue injury and regeneration. Cardiology and Cardiovascular Medicine. 2023;**7**(1):5-16. DOI: 10.26502/fccm.92920302

[23] Kandhwal M, Behl T, Singh S, Sharma N, Arora S, Bhatia S, et al. Role of matrix metalloproteinase in wound healing. American Journal of Translational Research. 2022;**14**(7):4391-4405

[24] Guo S, Dipietro LA. Factors affecting wound healing. Journal of Dental Research. 2010;**89**(3):219-229. DOI: 10.1177/0022034509359125

[25] Adair TH, Montani JP. Chapter 1, Overview of angiogenesis. In: Angiogenesis. San Rafael (CA): Morgan & Claypool Life Sciences; 2010. Available from: https://www.ncbi.nlm.nih.gov/books/NBK53238/

[26] Page MJ, Kell DB, Pretorius E. The role of lipopolysaccharide-induced cell signalling in chronic inflammation. Chronic Stress (Thousand Oaks). 2022;**6**:24705470221076390. DOI: 10.1177/24705470221076390

[27] Goswami AG, Basu S, Banerjee T, Shukla VK. Biofilm and wound healing: From bench to bedside. European Journal of Medical Research. 2023;**28**(1):157. DOI: 10.1186/s40001-023-01121-7

[28] Dolmatova EV, Wang K, Mandavilli R, Griendling KK. The effects of sepsis on endothelium and clinical implications. Cardiovascular Research. 2021;**117**(1):60-73. DOI: 10.1093/cvr/cvaa070

[29] Schilrreff P, Alexiev U. Chronic inflammation in non-healing skin wounds and promising natural bioactive compounds treatment. International Journal of Molecular Sciences. 2022;**23**(9):4928. DOI: 10.3390/ijms23094928

[30] Altalbawy FMA, Mukhlif BAM, Hussen A. Regenerative potential of PRP-based scaffolds in chronic wound healing: Mechanisms, advances, and therapeutic insights. Regenerative Therapy. 2025;**30**:278-298. DOI: 10.1016/j.reth.2025.06.008

[31] Empitu MA, Kadariswantiningsih IN, Shakri NM. Pharmacological strategies for targeting biofilms in otorhinolaryngologic infections and overcoming antimicrobial resistance (review). Biomedical Reports. 2025;**22**(6):95. DOI: 10.3892/br.2025.1973

[32] Patel S, Srivastava S, Singh MR. Mechanistic insight into diabetic wounds: Pathogenesis, molecular targets and treatment strategies to pace wound healing. Biomedicine and Pharmacotherapy. 2019;**112**:0753-3322. DOI: 10.1016/j.biopha.2019.108615

[33] Manna B, Nahirniak P, Morrison CA. Wound debridement. In: StatPearls [Internet]. Treasure Island (FL): StatPearls Publishing; 2025. Available from: https://www.ncbi.nlm.nih.gov/books/NBK507882/

[34] Fu K, Zheng X, Chen Y. Role of matrix metalloproteinases in diabetic foot ulcers: Potential therapeutic targets. Frontiers in Pharmacology. 2022;**13**. DOI: 10.3389/fphar.2022.1050630

[35] Li S, Renick P, Senkowsky J, Nair A, Tang L. Diagnostics for wound infections. Advances in wound care (New Rochelle). 2021;**10**(6):317-327. DOI: 10.1089/wound.2019.1103

[36] Sharma S, Mohler J, Mahajan SD, Schwartz SA, Bruggemann L, Aalinkeel R. Microbial biofilm: A review on formation, infection, antibiotic resistance, control measures, and innovative treatment. Microorganisms. 2023;**11**(6):1614. DOI: 10.3390/microorganisms11061614

[37] Veith AP, Henderson K, Spencer A, Sligar AD, Baker AB. Therapeutic strategies for enhancing angiogenesis in wound healing. Advanced Drug Delivery Reviews. 2019;**146**:97-125. DOI: 10.1016/j.addr.2018.09.010

[38] Gibson DJ, Schultz GS. Molecular wound assessments: Matrix metalloproteinases. Advances in wound care (New Rochelle). 2013;**2**(1):18-23. DOI: 10.1089/wound.2011.0359

[39] Larkins MC, Thombare A. Point-of-care testing. In: StatPearls [Internet]. Treasure Island (FL): StatPearls Publishing; 2025. Available from: https://www.ncbi.nlm.nih.gov/books/NBK592387/

[40] Binnie A, Lage J, Dos Santos CC. How can biomarkers be used to differentiate between infection and non-infectious causes of inflammation? In: Evidence-Based Practice of Critical Care. 2020. pp. 319-324.e1. DOI: 10.1016/B978-0-323-64068-8.00055-9

[41] Leboueny M, Maloupazoa Siawaya AC, Bouanga LDJ, Mvoundza Ndjindji O, Mveang Nzoghe A, Djoba Siawaya JF. Changes of C-reactive protein and Procalcitonin after four weeks of treatment in patients with pulmonary TB. Journal of Clinical Tuberculosis and Other Mycobacterial Diseases. 2023;**31**:100348. DOI: 10.1016/j.jctube.2023.100348

[42] Dai X, Shen L. Advances and trends in omics technology development.

Frontiers in Medicine. 2022;**9**:911861. DOI: 10.3389/fmed.2022.911861

[43] O'Brien J, Hayder H, Zayed Y, Peng C. Overview of microRNA biogenesis, mechanisms of actions, and circulation. Frontiers in Endocrinology. 2018;**9**:402. DOI: 10.3389/fendo.2018.00402

[44] Soliman AM, Das S, Abd Ghafar N, Teoh SL. Role of microRNA in proliferation phase of wound healing. Frontiers in Genetics. 2018;**9**:38. DOI: 10.3389/fgene.2018.00038

[45] Mulholland EJ, Dunne N, McCarthy HO. MicroRNA as therapeutic targets for chronic wound healing. Molecular Therapy - Nucleic Acids. 2017;**8**:46-55. DOI: 10.1016/j.omtn.2017.06.003

[46] Fakouri A, Razavi ZS, Mohammed AT, Hussein AHA, Afkhami H, Hooshiar MH. Applications of mesenchymal stem cell-exosome components in wound infection healing: New insights. Burns & Trauma. 2024;**12**. DOI: 10.1093/burnst/tkae021

[47] Wang Z, Zhao F, Xu C, Zhang Q, Ren H, Huang X, et al. Metabolic reprogramming in skin wound healing. Burns. Trauma. 2024;**12**:tkad047. DOI: 10.1093/burnst/tkad047

[48] Bao P, Kodra A, Tomic-Canic M, Golinko MS, Ehrlich HP, Brem H. The role of vascular endothelial growth factor in wound healing. The Journal of Surgical Research. 2009;**153**(2):347-358. DOI: 10.1016/j.jss.2008.04.023

[49] Saadh MJ, Jasim NY, Ahmed MH, Ballal S, Kumar A, Atteri S, et al. Critical roles of miR-21 in promotions angiogenesis: Friend or foe? Clinical and Experimental Medicine. 2025;**25**(1):66. DOI: 10.1007/s10238-025-01600-7

[50] Harmanci D, Erkan EP, Kocak A, Akdogan GG. Role of the microRNA-29 family in fibrotic skin diseases. Biomedical Reports. 2017;**6**(6):599-604. DOI: 10.3892/br.2017.900

[51] Sung BH, Parent CA, Weaver AM. Extracellular vesicles: Critical players during cell migration. Developmental Cell. 2021;**56**(13):1861-1874. DOI: 10.1016/j.devcel.2021.03.020

[52] Zeng QL, Liu DW. Mesenchymal stem cell-derived exosomes: An emerging therapeutic strategy for normal and chronic wound healing. World Journal of Clinical Cases. 2021;**9**(22):6218-6233. DOI: 10.12998/wjcc.v9.i22.6218

[53] Piipponen M, Li D, Landén NX. The immune functions of keratinocytes in skin wound healing. International Journal of Molecular Sciences. 2020;**21**(22):8790. DOI: 10.3390/ijms21228790

[54] Li P, Hong G, Zhan W, Deng M, Tu C, Wei J, et al. Endothelial progenitor cell derived exosomes mediated miR-182-5p delivery accelerate diabetic wound healing via down-regulating PPARG. International Journal of Medical Sciences. 2023;**20**(4):468-481. DOI: 10.7150/ijms.78790

[55] Zhang R, Li M, Li H, Ran X, Jin F, Tan Q, et al. Immune cell-derived exosomes in inflammatory disease and inflammatory tumor microenvironment: A review. Journal of Inflammation Research. 2024;**17**. DOI: 10.2147/JIR.S421649

[56] Bhandari R, Yang H, Kosarek NN, Smith AE, Garlick JA, Hinchcliff M, et al. Human dermal fibroblast-derived exosomes induce macrophage activation in systemic sclerosis. Rheumatology (Oxford, England).

2023;**62**(SI):SI114-SI124. DOI: 10.1093/rheumatology/keac453

[57] Hade MD, Suire CN, Suo Z. Mesenchymal stem cell-derived exosomes: Applications in regenerative medicine. Cells. 2021;**10**(8):1959. DOI: 10.3390/cells10081959

[58] Sun T, Li M, Liu Q, Yu A, Cheng K, Ma J, et al. Insights into optimizing exosome therapies for acute skin wound healing and other tissue repair. Frontiers in Medicine. 2024;**18**(2):258-284. DOI: 10.1007/s11684-023-1031-9

[59] Qiu S, Cai Y, Yao H, Lin C, Xie Y, Tang S, et al. Small molecule metabolites: Discovery of biomarkers and therapeutic targets. Signal Transduction and Targeted Therapy. 2023;**8**(1):132. DOI: 10.1038/s41392-023-01399-3

[60] Junka A, Wojtowicz W, Ząbek A, Krasowski G, Smutnicka D, Bakalorz B, et al. Metabolic profiles of exudates from chronic leg ulcerations. Journal of Pharmaceutical and Biomedical Analysis. 2017;**137**:13-22. DOI: 10.1016/j.jpba.2017.01.018

[61] Xiong Y, Knoedler S, Alfertshofer M, Kim BS, Jiang D, Liu G, et al. Mechanisms and therapeutic opportunities in metabolic aberrations of diabetic wounds: A narrative review. Cell Death & Disease. 2025;**16**(1):341. DOI: 10.1038/s41419-025-07583-3

[62] Baddam S, Tubben RE. Lactic acidosis. In: StatPearls [Internet]. Treasure Island (FL): StatPearls Publishing; 2025. Available from: https://www.ncbi.nlm.nih.gov/books/NBK470202/

[63] Kalkhof S, Förster Y, Schmidt J, Schulz MC, Baumann S, Weißflog A, et al. Proteomics and metabolomics for in situ monitoring of wound healing. BioMed Research International. 2014;**2014**:934848. DOI: 10.1155/2014/934848

[64] Gobena S, Admassu B, Kinde MZ, Gessese AT. Proteomics and its current application in biomedical area: Concise review. The Scientific World Journal. 2024;**2024**:4454744. DOI: 10.1155/2024/4454744

[65] Johnson KE, Wilgus TA. Vascular endothelial growth factor and angiogenesis in the regulation of cutaneous wound repair. Advances in wound care (New Rochelle). 2014;**3**(10):647-661. DOI: 10.1089/wound.2013.0517

[66] Deng Z, Fan T, Xiao C, et al. TGF-β signaling in health, disease and therapeutics. Signal Transduction and Targeted Therapy. 2024;**9**:61. DOI: 10.1038/s41392-024-01764-w

[67] Caley MP, Martins VL, O'Toole EA. Metalloproteinases and wound healing. Advances in wound care (New Rochelle). 2015;**4**(4):225-234. DOI: 10.1089/wound.2014.0581

[68] Mahmoud NN, Hamad K, Al Shibitini A, Juma S, Sharifi S, Gould L, et al. Investigating inflammatory markers in wound healing: Understanding implications and identifying artifacts. ACS Pharmacology & Translational Science. 2024;**7**(1):18-27. DOI: 10.1021/acsptsci.3c00336

[69] Franz S, Torregrossa M, Anderegg U. Dysregulated S100A9 expression impairs matrix deposition in chronic wounds. International Journal of Molecular Sciences. 2024;**25**(18):9980. DOI: 10.3390/ijms25189980

[70] Cialdai F, Risaliti C, Monici M. Role of fibroblasts in wound healing

and tissue remodeling on Earth and in space. Frontiers in Bioengineering and Biotechnology. 2022;**10**:958381. DOI: 10.3389/fbioe.2022.958381

[71] Şimşek T, Şimşek HU, Cantürk NZ. Response to trauma and metabolic changes: Posttraumatic metabolism. Ulusal Cerrahi Dergisi. 2014;**30**(3):153-159. DOI: 10.5152/UCD.2014.2653

Section 2

Clinical Evaluation and Therapeutic Decision-Making

Chapter 2

Therapeutic Advances in Chronic Wound Management: A Review of Debridement Strategies and Emerging Approaches

Jorge Adrián Garza-Cerna, Gabriel Ángel Mecott-Rivera, Eugenia Paris Coronado, Yanko Castro-Govea, José Juan Pérez-Trujillo, Roberto Montes de Oca-Luna, Daniel Salas-Treviño, Guadalupe Tirma González-Mateo, Valeria Kopytina and Jorge López Berroa

Abstract

Chronic wounds significantly impact health, diminishing the quality of life for patients and caregivers. These conditions demand substantial financial and time resources from medical teams and are often complicated by comorbidities. The following chapter raises awareness of social costs concerning chronic wounds while reviewing the most recent knowledge and strategies regarding the clinical approach to improve healing outcomes and treatment adherence. Here, traditional and innovative chronic wound management techniques are examined, including wound bed care, dressings, antibiotic therapy, and advanced debridement methods. Special focus is given to debridement due to its critical role in wound healing and functional recovery. Collagenase, a widely used enzymatic debridement agent, selectively degrades denatured collagen while preserving healthy tissue, promoting effective wound cleaning and healing. Exposing healthy tissue enhances the efficacy of complementary treatments and accelerates recovery. Therefore, targeted debridement methods are pivotal in chronic wound management, improving healing and patient outcomes. Identifying critical barriers such as wound stalling, infection, and ischemia, as well as understanding factors that influence adherence and implementing patient-specific interventions, is equally vital. Innovations in wound care formulations designed to enhance comfort, reduce infection risk, and promote faster healing are essential for improving both adherence and quality of life in chronic wound patients.

Keywords: debridement, chronic ulcers, chronic wounds, collagenase, wound healing, wound care therapies, vascularization, wound stalling, edge management

1. Introduction

Chronic wounds are lesions that are not resolved through a normal healing process within the expected timeframe. The natural repair process starts with an inflammatory reaction, releasing cytokines that trigger a proliferative phase during which new tissue, blood vessels, and extracellular matrix (ECM) are formed. Afterward, the wound shrinks as the ECM is remodeled. However, chronic or excessive inflammation disrupts the process, turning it pathological and potentially hindering healing or causing excess ECM [1].

Managing chronic wounds is complex, requiring prolonged treatments and often involving multidisciplinary therapies to address underlying causes, symptoms, and complications. This scenario increases the burden on the healthcare system and complicates clinical decisions, underscoring the need for efficient strategies [2].

Apart from economic cost, chronic wounds also pose a significant challenge to public health due to a profound impact on patient quality of life, together with a loss of productivity. Chronic wounds impact the quality of life of nearly 2.5% of the United States population [3]. Studies published between 2016 and 2019 estimated that chronic wounds account for approximately 1–5.5% of the total healthcare expenditure in developed countries [2].

In the past decade, over US$25 billion was spent each year on the treatment of chronic wounds, and it was projected that 1–2% of people will suffer from a chronic wound at some point in their lives in developed countries [2, 4].

Chronic wounds represent a silent but widespread epidemic that impacts a significant segment of the global population and generates biological, psychological, social, and financial issues for both patients and the healthcare system. Therefore, there is a critical need to develop more effective treatments that can reduce healing times, complications, and costs.

It is important to highlight that the challenge of treating chronic wounds is intensifying, propelled by an aging population and a notable increase in chronic diseases such as diabetes and obesity rates across the globe [3].

This review examines various available approaches for chronic wounds including wound bed care, debridement treatments, skin dressings, and antibiotic therapy, and discusses potential improvements specifically in debridement options, a crucial step in these healing and functional restoration processes.

2. Chronic wound development, associated complications, and assessment

2.1 Overview of wound healing phases

Wound healing is a dynamic and complex process that involves four overlapping phases, including hemostasis, which initiates coagulation to stop bleeding; inflammation, where recruitment of immune cells is promoted in order to control infection; proliferation, which involves the formation of granulation tissue and angiogenesis; and remodeling, characterized by collagen maturation and wound contraction [5]. Any disruption in these stages can result in wound stalling, often observed in chronic wounds, requiring timely intervention to resume progression.

The role of immune cells is crucial throughout these stages. Inflammation is a necessary and self-limited stage (in normal conditions) characterized by the influx of inflammatory cells to the wound area. During proliferation, connective and granulation tissue fills the wound, supported by the growth of keratinocytes, fibroblasts, and endothelial cells. Then, a resurfacing process involves the migration of epithelial cells from the wound edges across the granulation tissue, leading to the restoration of the skin barrier. Granulation tissue formation is crucial for wound healing, as it provides the ECM and microvascular foundation for re-epithelialization [6].

Tissue-resident cells and infiltrating leukocytes promote angiogenesis by secreting factors like VEGF, TGF-β1, and IL8. Vascular formation occurs through sprouting from existing endothelial cells, supplemented by other cell types transitioning into endothelial roles. In addition, neutrophils have been recognized to participate in angiogenesis during later stages. This process is regulated by a balance of proangiogenic and antiangiogenic factors, ensuring proper vascularization [6].

The remodeling phase involves the reorganization of collagen fibers and the gradual contraction of wound edges, driven by increasing tensile strength, leading to the restoration of tissue integrity. Optimal healing should occur with minimal fibrosis, restoring the tissue to its original state as the scarless process in fetal tissues, characterized by an efficient regeneration due to a high ratio of regenerative to inflammatory cells, limited inflammatory response, and different ECM composition compared to adults. However, adult healing typically involves a fibrotic response, resulting in collagen-rich scar tissue [5].

2.2 Chronic wound development, associated complications, and assessment

Chronic wounds often become stalled in the inflammatory phase of healing, a phenomenon referred to as wound stalling. This interruption is frequently caused by an imbalance in proteolytic activity, persistent low-grade bacterial colonization, excessive fibrin deposition, or underlying systemic conditions such as diabetes mellitus or vascular insufficiency. When the repair process remains unresolved in the inflammatory phase, it triggers an excessive, pathological, and damaging immune response. Persistent inflammation continuously releases inflammatory cytokines, proteases, and free radicals, which degrade growth factors and ECM needed for repair. Likewise, it prevents the proliferation of key cells for regeneration and wound closure such as fibroblasts and keratinocytes [6].

Another key impediment to epithelial resurfacing is the development of a smooth, hardened, sclerotic wound bed resulting from aberrant tissue remodeling, a process that can be likened to eburnation observed in bone lesions. This sclerotic surface inhibits epithelial cell migration, ultimately preventing re-epithelialization [7].

Typically, chronic wounds are those that do not follow an orderly and timely process to achieve anatomical and functional restoration and, after at least 4 weeks, still show no signs of progressive healing. This is a benchmark to differentiate chronic from acute wounds, which usually show signs of healing within a shorter, more predictable timeframe [8].

Healing disruption can be triggered by metabolic or pathological factors, such as diabetes (in diabetic foot lesions), cutaneous fragility (e.g., Epidermolysis bullosa, rare skin disorders where chronic wounds arise spontaneously or following minor physical trauma), vascular (arterial or venous), neuropathic, rheumatological diseases as well as local factors such as sustained pressure, infection, and microbial biofilms, edema, or even pharmacological treatments [9]. Chronic wounds can result also from iatrogenic and external causes including surgery, burns, traumatism, or complications from acute wounds. Contributing factors such as chronic hypoxia, age, obesity, smoking, mobility deficits, immunodeficiency, poor nutrition, and vitamin status [10] are also remarkable. Moreover, non-viable tissue, foreign bodies, and improper moisture levels also participate in the process (**Figure 1**) [9].

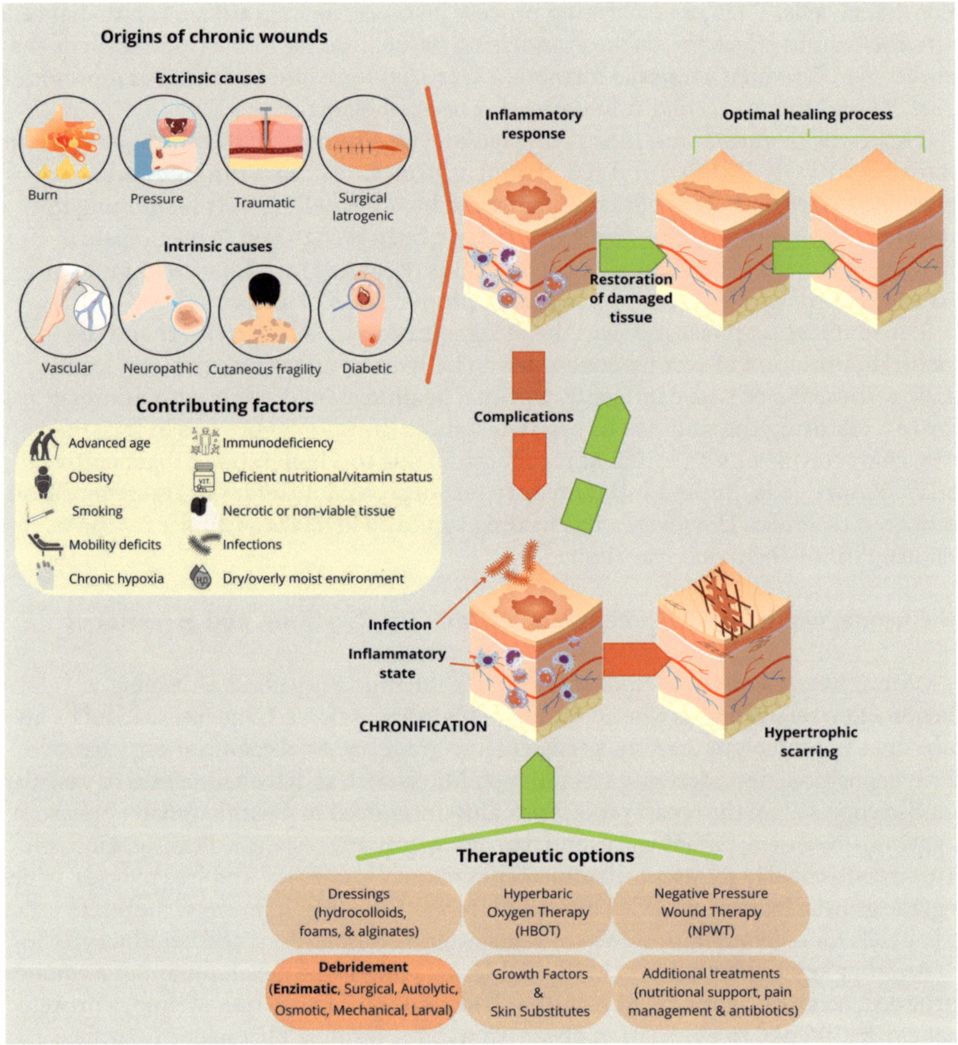

Figure 1.
Healing dynamics, causes, and contributing factors of chronic wounds. This process normally involves a necessary inflammatory reaction to eliminate pathogens, clear debris, and initiate tissue repair, followed by a proliferation phase and a maturation stage. Optimal wound healing aims for closure without fibrous scarring and restoration of integrity. The disruption of the normal healing process leads to sustained inflammation. This sustained inflammatory environment prevents the wound from progressing through the natural healing stages, keeping it in a constant state of injury and repair, and thus, becoming a chronic wound, for which different therapeutic options are available.

Each type of chronic wound has distinct characteristics and contributing factors, such as pressure-induced ischemia in pressure ulcers or impaired glucose control in diabetic ulcers [4].

2.3 Diagnosis, assessment, and challenges

Visual examination, wound swabbing, and biopsies are employed techniques alongside diagnostic imaging to understand wound extent and underlying pathologies, to achieve an accurate diagnosis, and to select optimal therapeutic interventions [11].

Infection is a common complication associated with chronic wounds, causing a significant hurdle in the management of these conditions [12].

Another major challenge is scarring, which can have profound functional and esthetic consequences, affecting the patient's psychological well-being.

Moreover, wounds can lead to further complications, such as Marjolin's ulcers, an uncommon skin cancer, often diagnosed during the evaluation of lesions within persistent wounds like pressure sores or leg ulcers, occurring in 1–2% of burn scars [10].

3. Chronic wound treatments

Conventional treatments for chronic wounds focus on wound bed preparation, essential for healing, including sanitization, necrotic tissue removal, moisture management with appropriate dressings, inflammation control using anti-inflammatory agents, and infection prevention through antibiotics, antiseptics, and proper hygiene [12, 13]. These conventional approaches have been continuously refined, leading to the development of more effective strategies, including debridement, advanced dressings, negative pressure, hyperbaric oxygen therapy, growth factors, skin substitutes, and others such as nanofat or biocellular therapies (**Table 1**). Moreover, adjunctive approaches improve healing outcomes.

The condition of wound edges plays a crucial prognostic role in the healing of chronic wounds (**Figure 2**). Nonprogressive or rolled edges (epibole) indicate arrested epithelial migration and require debridement or marginal stimulation to resume healing. Necrotic or devitalized margins, which are often black or yellow and adherent, significantly delay healing and increase the risk of infection if not promptly debrided. Macerated edges appear white and brittle due to excess moisture, hinder epithelialization, and require moisture regulation. Hyperkeratotic or calloused edges, which are common in diabetic foot ulcers, prevent closure unless mechanically or surgically removed. Conversely, viable and progressive epithelial margins, characterized by a thin, pink, and slightly raised margin with a visible epithelial tongue, are associated with favorable healing outcomes and faster closure. To prevent chronicity and optimize the healing process, regular check-ups and targeted interventions at the wound edges are essential [27, 28].

3.1 Adjunctive approaches in chronic wound management

Supportive measures such as nutritional optimization and pain management play a crucial role in enhancing overall treatment outcomes. Regarding nutritional support, it is important to highlight that an adequate protein intake, along with vitamins and minerals provides substrates and co-factors for cell-mediated support healing.

Analgesics to manage discomfort and reduce the likeness of scratching and subsequent physical damage are crucial for pain management. Topical creams, gels, or patches containing analgesics can be applied directly over the wound for pain relief [29].

3.2 Debridement treatments

Debridement is the standard care to prepare wounds for proper healing since it removes non-viable tissues, reduces bacterial load, controls the inflammatory environment, promotes healthy granulation tissue, creates a uniform bed for eventual grafting or application of dressing, and prevents traumatic scarring [14].

Type	Subtypes & basis	Pros	Cons	Regimen & times	Refs
Surgical debridement	Surgery	• Rapid removal of necrotic tissue • Precise control over the area • Immediate	• Requires skilled practitioners. • Needs anesthesia. • Risk of infection • Not for all patients	From few minutes to 1 h, depending on wound extent. Healing takes weeks to months	[14]
Autolytic debridement	Uses the body's own enzymes and moisture to liquefy dead tissue.	• Gentle, non-invasive • Uses body's own enzymes. • Safe for healthy tissue	• Slow process • Not effective for heavily infected wounds • Requires moisture-retentive dressings	Slow, as it relies on the body's own mechanisms. Can take several days to weeks to show results	[15]
Osmotic debridement	Uses hypertonic systems, like sugar or honey, which help draw fluid from the wound to the surface.	Reduces edema and softens hard eschar and slough Dehydrate bacteria	• Can cause pain/discomfort. • Lacks antimicrobial properties. • Can be expensive. • Excess moisture cause maceration	Requires a few days	[16]
Mechanical debridement	Wet-to-dry dressings, irrigation, hydrotherapy, and scrubbing.	• Cost-effective • Effective for wounds with large exudate	• Can be painful. • Risk of damaging new tissue • Less selective • Costly material	Relatively quick in removing dead tissue but may need several repetitions over days to weeks	[17]
Larval debridement	*Lucilia sericata* fly maggots that release enzymes to liquefy dead tissue & ingest it	• Highly selective • Clean slough & infection • Access hard-to-reach areas	• Availability can be an issue • Psychological dis-comfort – Careful monitoring	Can take several days to a week. The overall healing requires additional weeks to months	[12]

DOI: http://dx.doi.org/10.5772/intechopen.1011088

Type	Subtypes & basis	Pros	Cons	Regimen & times	Refs
Enzymatic debridement	Collagenase, Chymotrypsin/ Trypsin, Papain, Fibrinolysin, Streptokinase/ Streptodornase	• Selective for necrotic tissue • Combinable with other methods • Less painful and faster than others	• Can be expensive. • Risk of allergic reactions • Depends on wound milieu	Faster than others like autolytic debridement. It may take a few days to weeks	[18–20]
Advanced dressings	Hydrocolloid, Foam, Alginate. Maintain a moist environment. Do not remove necrotic tissue	• Moist environment • Bacterial protection • Absorbent • Less frequent changes than traditional dressing	• Hydrocolloids are not indicated for heavy exudates. • Maceration risks • Residue issues • Foam and alginate not for dry wounds	Remains for up to a week before change is needed. Healing times range from weeks to months	[21]
Negative pressure therapy	Draw out fluid from the wound and contract the edges.	• Reduces edema and bacterial load. • Promotes granulation. • Reduces healing time & scarring	• Specialized equipment needed. • Costly • Present contraindications	Several weeks to months, with changes in the dressing system typically two to three times per week	[22]
Hyperbaric oxygen therapy	Increases the oxygen supply, improving healing & reducing infection risks.	• Increases oxygen in blood. • Fights infection • Improves circulation	• Expensive • Specialized facilities needed • Present contraindications	Multiple sessions (daily or several times a week) over several weeks or months	[23]

Type	Subtypes & basis	Pros	Cons	Regimen & times	Refs
Growth factors / skin substitutes	Growth factors stimulate cell proliferation.	• Promote tissue regeneration directly. • Reduce healing times	• Very expensive • Risk of rejection • Regulatory challenges • Continuous application and monitoring over months	May provide quicker initial responses in some wounds	[24, 25]
Nanofat	Adipose-derived stem cells, paracrine factors, exosomes & ECM components.	• Modulates inflammation • Promotes tissue regeneration	• Specialized equipment needed • Prolonged preparation time • Variable cell yield	Visible results within 1 to 2 weeks. Repeat applications may be needed	[26]
Biocellular therapies	stem or progenitor cells + bioactive components (PRP, PPP, or dermal matrices).	• Promote organized tissue regeneration • Replace damaged tissue	• Regulatory issues • High cost • Need for laboratory infrastructure	Highly individualized regimens. May involve one or more applications over weeks to months	[26]

Table 1.
Comparison treatment approaches for chronic wounds. Pros, Cons, times of treatment, and subtypes for chronic wound approaches.

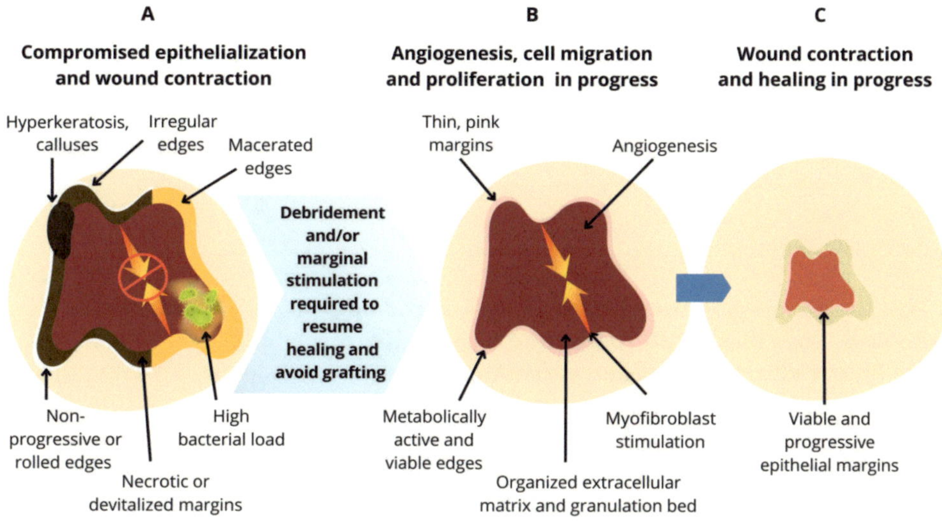

Figure 2.
Impact of wound margin conditions on wound contracture. Debridement may serve as an effective approach to stimulate the wound edge, with the aim of reinitiating the healing process and avoiding the need for grafting.

Depending on the clinical situation, type of wound, presence of infection, patient tolerance, and desired outcome, strategies include surgical, autolytic, osmotic, mechanical, larval or enzymatic debridement (**Table 1**).

3.2.1 Surgical or sharp debridement

Surgical debridement is a traditional intervention, accepted as the fastest and most selective approach, being the preferred method in cases of extensive necrosis, heavy bacterial load or advanced infection, adherent slough, dry eschar, or deep pressure ulcers. Although bleeding may occur, it can be controlled using several methods. One risk of this technique is pain, especially in neuropathy patients who may present hyperesthesia and be more sensitive, and anesthesia is often required [30].

This method can be done by only removing the affected tissue or also adjacent healthy tissue to stimulate repair from uninvolved areas, reactivating granulation, and epithelialization. Therefore, this technique allows precise excision of selected tissue down to well-perfused viable planes [14].

This approach is highly valuable to prepare clean, non-irregular wound margins—free from maceration, hyperkeratosis, or nonprogressive tissue—which are metabolically active and capable of supporting effective epithelial migration from the edges toward the center of the wound. Surgical debridement, therefore, enhances wound edge viability, which is essential for enabling and sustaining the healing process (**Figure 2**). The ECM reorganizes, and wound contraction is facilitated by myofibroblasts. The ultimate aim of this procedure is spontaneous wound closure by epithelialization, avoiding skin grafting [27].

3.2.2 Autolytic debridement

This technique uses the body's proteolytic enzymes to liquefy dead tissue, therefore being a non-invasive and selective option, preserving healthy tissue. Dressings that maintain moisture (e.g., hydrocolloids and hydrogels) are used to facilitate this process driven by phagocytic cells and create an environment capable of liquefying slough and promoting granulation [15, 31].

Epithelialization proceeds centripetally from the preserved wound edges. This method maintains the integrity of basal dermal cells and local stem cell niches, which are essential for healing [31].

3.2.3 Osmotic debridement

The osmotic method contribute to gentle debridement by drawing moisture from devitalized tissue thanks to hypertonic dressings, like crystalline sugar or medical-grade honey, reducing edema and softening hard eschar and slough. This method also dehydrates bacterial cells, leading to their death [16].

Honey is one of the oldest known wound care substances, with documented use dating back to ancient civilizations. In recent decades, it has been re-evaluated by modern medicine and supported by extensive *in vitro* studies, preclinical models, and clinical trials. Its antimicrobial effects—particularly in medical-grade honey—support infection control. Moreover, recent evidence suggests that honey may exert immunomodulatory effects, helping to regulate inflammation and stimulate a more advantageous healing environment [32].

3.2.4 Mechanical debridement

This approach involves the physical removal of necrotic tissue or biofilm using abrasive materials, hydraulic forces, or friction-based techniques. This can be done using wet-to-dry dressings, where saline-moistened gauze is allowed to dry and adhere to the necrotic tissue; upon removal, the tissue is pulled away [17].

Other methods include monofilament dressings, pressurized irrigation, hydrotherapy, and scrubbing [17]. While effective, they are non-selective and may disrupt viable tissue if improperly applied.

3.2.5 Larval therapy

Also named maggot therapy, this technique uses sterile larvae of the green bottle fly, *Lucilia sericata*, which releases enzymes that specifically liquefy dead tissue to ingest it. Additionally, the larvae have antimicrobial effects and promote granulation tissue formation. The technique is highly precise and does not harm healthy tissue [15].

FDA-approved in 2004, this technique is particularly useful in patients with diabetic foot ulcers and other chronic wounds where surgical debridement is contraindicated or poorly tolerated. It is also employed when other debridement techniques have failed or are insufficient [33].

3.2.6 Enzymatic debridement

Enzymatic debridement applies exogenous proteolytic enzymes to digest non-viable, necrotic tissue [18].

Several aspects enhance enzymatic versus other debridement methods. First, its selectiveness for devitalized tissue avoids damaging newly formed granulation tissue, which is crucial for good healing and reduced scarring. Second, it is less invasive and can be performed with minimal discomfort to the patient compared to surgical debridement, which is quick but painful and requires anesthesia [19]. This makes it particularly useful for patients for whom surgery is too risky. Third, it is gentle and maintains a controlled removal of necrotic tissue [34], allowing effective granulation and eventually minimizing scarring. Finally, it can be easily combined with other strategies like dressings, negative pressure therapy, or even other debridement techniques [35]. This versatility ensures that the process can be tailored to the specific needs of the wound and patient, improving outcomes (**Figure 3**).

The selection of the enzymatic agent is crucial and depends on wound characteristics and the patient's condition. Different products are available containing collagenase, chymotrypsin/trypsin, fibrinolysin, papain combined with urea, subtilisin, and streptokinase-streptodornase combination [36].

Collagenase in ointment form is the most widely used enzymatic debrider. Derived primarily from *Clostridium histolyticum*, collagenase enables the preparation of the wound bed by breaking collagen bridges. Collagenase facilitates the removal of debris obstructing healing, reduces bacterial load, promotes a healthier environment for regeneration, and enables dermal cell migration and re-epithelialization [37]. This also prevents apoptosis and inflammation, contributing to a more conducive healing

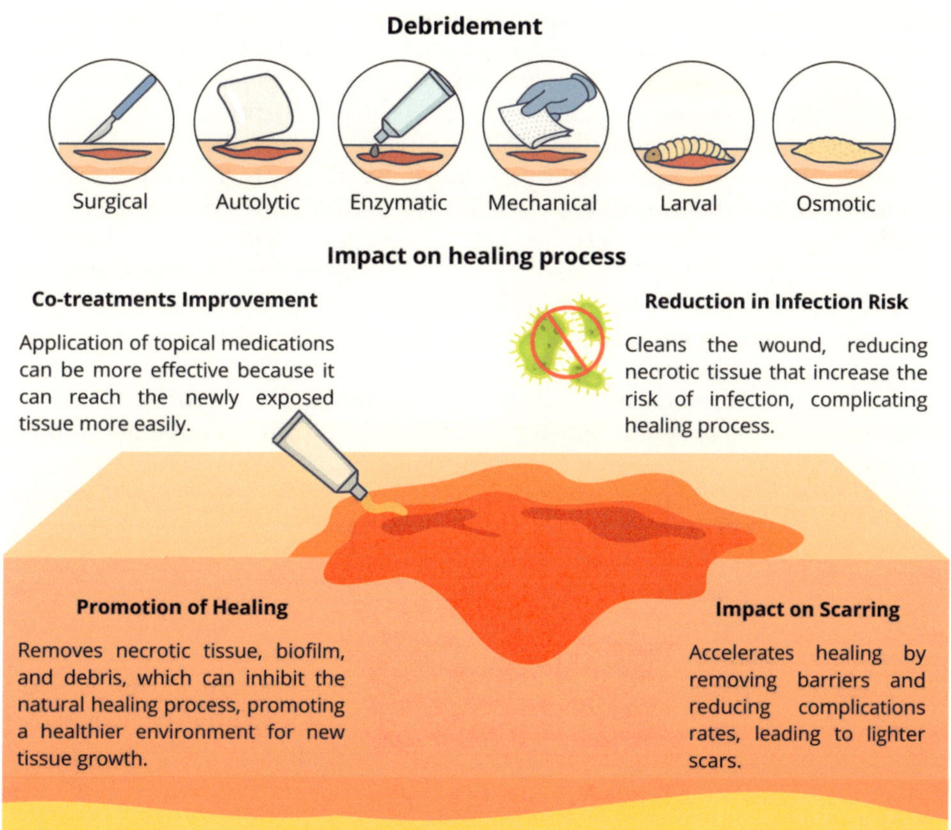

Figure 3.
Debridement options and impact on healing process. Debridement promotes healing, reduces infection risks, improves co-treatments, and reduces complications, leading to less scarring.

environment [38]. Moreover, collagenase shows good tolerability and a high rate of treatment adherence among patients [39] and showed positive results for burns and chronic ulcers [38].

A study in pediatric burns demonstrated the high effectiveness of topical collagenase, supporting outpatient management without long-term consequences and minimizing invasive interventions [40].

Recent studies highlight collagenase's role in managing acute burns, not only as a debriding agent but also potentially accelerating healing [41, 42]. Despite lacking antimicrobial activity, collagenase does not increase risks of infections compared to silver-impregnated products, the gold standard for non-antibiotic bacteriostatic management. Specifically, collagenase showed benefits in preventing burn depth conversion and reducing the need for surgeries, which may help offset its higher initial cost by decreasing the requirement for invasive treatments [41]. This is particularly advantageous since non-surgically managing deep burns can reduce morbidity and improve cosmetic and functional outcomes.

Unlike non-selective agents, collagenase preserves the integrity of growth factors and granulation tissue, which is crucial for healing [38]. This specificity also avoids unintended effects on the surrounding healthy tissue, minimizing costs and complications [43].

Different collagenase-based formulations are available. Collagenase Santyl® (Smith & Nephew) is a widely used product in ointment presentation that has been a prescribed treatment for over 50 years, indicating its established presence in wound care. Other commercialized products are Iruxol® (Smith & Nephew), Novuxol® or Noruxol® (Smith & Nephew), Bionect Start® (FIDIA Pharmaceutical), and Ulcoderma® (Smith & Nephew) [44, 45].

A retrospective observational study evaluated the efficacy of a hyaluronic acid and collagenase-based ointment (Bionect Start®) in 70 chronic wounds of varying etiologies, including diabetes, post-traumatic ulcers, burns, and pressure ulcers [42]. Results showed reduced healing time, improved healing quality, high satisfaction rates, and decreased patient-reported pain.

Ointment formulation is chosen to maintain the stability and activity of collagenase. Microemulsions offer greater product stability compared to gels. Of note, there is an ongoing study aiming to deepen the benefits of this presentation (data not published), using pbserum SHS30® (Proteos Biotech, S.L.), a novel microemulsion combining recombinant collagenases G and H (PB220), and a hyaluronate lyase (PB72K). This combination represents a new approach that, in addition to the activity of collagenase, promotes the reduction in the viscosity of biological fluids by the hyaluronate lyase, increasing vascular permeability and accessibility to the active ingredient [46]. The presence of r-Lyase acts by destabilizing the biofilm and preventing wound sepsis. Moreover, pbserum SHS30® novel single-dose format has the advantage of reducing the possibility of infections.

Another ongoing study is employing the combination of pbserum SHS30® with pbserum HA1.5 High® (Proteos Biotech, S.L.), an injectable solution composed of non-cross-linked high molecular weight hyaluronic acid mixed with lipase (PB500), collagenases G and H (PB220), and lyase (hyaluronidase, PB72K), with the goal of enhancing clinical outcomes. Hyaluronic acid has anti-inflammatory properties that can help reduce wound inflammation, contributing to faster and more effective healing. It also acts as a mechanical barrier (anti-adhesive gel), facilitating debridement in hypertrophic scars. Moreover, hyaluronic acid inhibits the upregulation of transforming growth factor beta (TGF-β), a key driver of fibrosis. This leads to a reduction in the inflammatory response within the wound—another contributing factor to fibrosis—and prevents the formation of disorganized collagen fibers, allowing them to realign and distribute in patterns resembling healthy tissue [47, 48]. **Figure 4** shows the evolution of two wounds treated with pbserum SHS30® and HA1.5 High®.

Debridement is commonly combined with antibiotics, but prolonged antibiotic use can cause side effects, requiring careful monitoring [49]. Silver sulfadiazine, an employed antimicrobial agent, can cause hypersensitivity and an exudate called pseudo-eschar, on the wound surface. Chloramphenicol, another employed agent (e.g, in Ulcoderma®), may lead to systemic effects (increased hematopoiesis) due to its absorption [50]. Moreover, an important percentage of patients treated with this combination require another antimicrobial agent [51].

Another problem associated with antimicrobial agents is the proteolytic activity within the wound environment, highly sensitive to pH levels. Collagenase operates optimally within a narrow pH range (6.0–8.0), which helps maintain its activity in degrading only non-viable components without harming surrounding viable tissue [52]. Chronic wounds tend to have a more alkaline pH (7.4–8.9) than healthy skin, which can inhibit healing by allowing destructive protease activities [53]. Adjusting the wound's pH to a more acidic environment could reduce protease activities, thereby fostering healing and collagenase efficacy. Antiseptic solutions notably affect the pH, reducing collagenase efficacy. Therefore, avoiding antiseptic solutions is interesting for maintaining this optimal pH. Products that do not include antibiotics in their formulation, such as pbserum SHS30®, do not present these drawbacks.

Treatment times and healing duration vary significantly based on wound type, size, patient comorbidities, and debridement method used. Surgical methods offer the fastest tissue clearance but may require multiple sessions. Autolytic and enzymatic techniques are slower, often requiring several days to weeks for full effect. Larval therapy can produce visible results in 3–4 days but may not be acceptable to all patients. Osmotic and mechanical techniques may require daily care and monitoring [54, 55].

3.3 Conventional and advanced dressings

While traditional dressings (such as dry gauze) are still used in some settings, other dressings such as hydrocolloids, foams, or alginates better maintain a moist environment conducive to healing and may support debridement when used as part of an integrated wound care strategy [21]. Smart bandages have been recently developed by using wireless technology to detect inflammation, infections, or problems with blood flow to alert patients and healthcare providers during real-time treatment [56]. These new technologies could potentially include bioelectronic materials to deliver electrical stimulation and incorporate advanced hydrogels [57]. In this regard, there is an ongoing clinical trial testing Exciflex (Ohio, USA), an electronic bandage with components of a stimulation system mounted on a flexible substrate [58].

3.4 Other emerging and recently developed treatments for chronic wounds

In parallel with conventional and moisture-retentive dressing strategies, more recent therapeutic approaches have emerged:

Negative pressure therapy facilitates wound healing by removing excess fluid and promoting wound edge contraction, thereby accelerating recovery and minimizing scarring. Its effectiveness is maximized when the wound bed is adequately prepared, often through debridement [22].

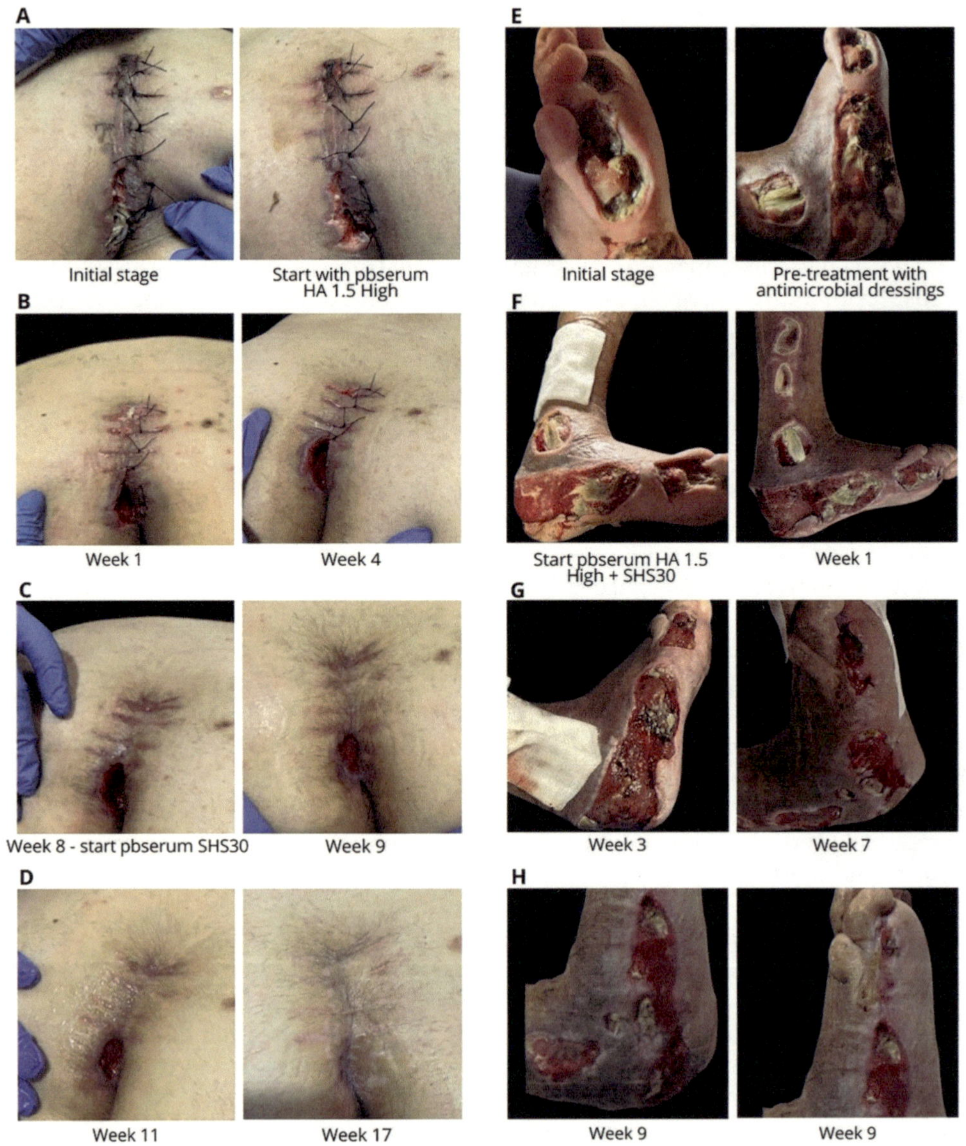

Figure 4.
Wound healing progression in two clinical cases using enzymatic therapy, combining pbserum SHS30 and HA1.5 high. Time is expressed in weeks from the initiation of enzymatic treatment. No grafting was performed in either case. Dressing changes were performed every 48 hours, with enzymatic applications maintained throughout the treatment period. (A–D) Sequential wound evolution in a 25-year-old female with a post-surgical soft tissue defect following pilonidal abscess and sepsis. The protocol included thorough irrigation with Anasept Antimicrobial Cleanser® (Anacapa Technologies, Inc., USA), followed by enzyme application, placement of Fibracol® (3 M Health Care, USA) collagen sheet, and closure with Omnifix® (Paul-Hartmann AG, Germany). (A) Initial wound dimensions: 3 cm deep, 3 cm long, and 2.2 cm wide. Following initial autolytic debridement with dressings for 2 weeks and six sessions of hyperbaric oxygen therapy, the patient started enzymatic debridement. (B) She received weekly pbserum HA 1.5 High irrigation. (C) From week 8 of enzymatic treatment, pbserum HA 1.5 High was combined with pbserum SHS30 applied twice weekly. (D) Progressive marginal re-epithelialization was observed, confirming effective peripheral-to-central closure without grafting. Complete closure was achieved after approximately 4 months (16 weeks). (E–H) Images correspond to a 97-year-old male with a pressure ulcer of 2 months of evolution. Prior to prescribing treatment, the wound was infected, with abundant purulent exudate, foul odor, and significant depth. Dimensions included lateral aspect of the foot, 24 × 4 cm; plantar area below the toes, 3 × 4 cm; and over the lateral malleolus, 6 × 4 cm. Irrigation with Anasept

Antimicrobial Cleanser® was initiated, followed by packing with Anasept Gel® and dressing changes every 48 hours, in combination with systemic antibiotic therapy. This approach enabled effective autolytic debridement. Two small bone fragments were surgically removed from the distal metatarsal region of the left foot and the plantar aspect. (E) Negative pressure wound therapy (VAC) was conducted, with dressing changes every 72 hours for two weeks. (F) Enzymatic therapy started on a 72-hour rotation: pbserum SHS30 applied one day and HA1.5 High on the next. Following enzyme application, Fibracol® collagen sheets and Cutimed Sorbact ® (Essity AB, Germany) mesh (with antimicrobial properties) were used to cover the wound bed. The area was then wrapped with a Klin bandage and an elastic compression bandage. A protective offloading boot was also applied to eliminate pressure over the wound site. (G) Clinical improvement was noted during the early phase of treatment, with new granulation tissue and reduction of macerated areas. Restoration of clean, non-hyperkeratotic wound margins was achieved, promoting early stages of marginal re-epithelialization. (H) Despite partial wound resolution, the patient died of acute myocardial infarction prior to complete closure. Enzymatic treatment was performed during 2.3 months (9 weeks). Nonetheless, wound edge activation and tissue organization were evident during follow-up.

Hyperbaric oxygen therapy increases the oxygen supply to the wound, enhancing healing and reducing risks of infections. This therapy is complementary to debridement [23].

Growth factors and skin substitutes promote tissue regeneration directly. This effect can be significantly hampered by the presence of necrotic tissue, highlighting the importance of debridement [24].

High-density platelet-rich plasma (HD-PRP) is an autologous concentrate of platelets obtained through blood centrifugation. It contains a high concentration of growth factors such as PDGF, VEGF, TGF-β, and EGF, which promote angiogenesis, fibroblast migration, cell proliferation, and collagen synthesis. In chronic wound management, HD-PRP accelerates granulation tissue formation, reduces inflammation, and creates a more favorable environment for re-epithelialization.

Platelet-poor plasma (PPP) is the plasma fraction with a low platelet count, often discarded. However, recent evidence supports its use due to the presence of fibrinogen and plasma proteins, contributing to biological scaffolding, as well as its anti-inflammatory and hemostatic properties. PPP is used as a complementary agent to PRP or as a biological matrix combined with dressings or biomaterials, which is particularly useful in structurally deficient wounds.

Nanofat offers strong regenerative potential since it acts as a bio-stimulant, modulating inflammation and promoting tissue regeneration, even in poorly vascularized wound beds. Nanofat is derived from adipose tissue through emulsification and filtration, removing mature adipocytes while preserving adipose-derived stem cells, together with paracrine factors and exosomes as well as components of the ECM [26]. Typically applied after surgical or enzymatic debridement.

Biocellular therapies combine living cellular elements (e.g., stem or progenitor cells) with bioactive components such as PRP, PPP, or dermal matrices. Their goal is to modulate the wound microenvironment, promote organized tissue regeneration, and repair or replace damaged tissue [26].

4. Factors promoting healing

Several factors positively influence the wound healing process, including moisture balance and vascular integrity. In fact, a moist wound environment supports cell migration and autolytic debridement. Vascular integrity allows adequate arterial and venous circulation that ensures the supply of nutrients and the removal of waste. Also crucial is adequate oxygenation, which is needed for ATP production, collagen synthesis, angiogenesis, and bacterial defense [59].

It is well-known that granulation tissue is key for wound healing, as it provides the ECM and microvascular foundation for re-epithelialization. Impaired granulation, often due to poor perfusion or infection, requires targeted interventions to restore balance and support matrix deposition. Since successful wound management depends on sufficient tissue perfusion, non-invasive tools such as transcutaneous oxygen measurement (TcPO2), ankle-brachial index (ABI), and laser Doppler imaging can aid in assessing local vascularity and guiding therapeutic decisions [60, 61].

In the same way, correct nutritional status and glycemic control are essential for healing. Vitamin C, zinc, and arginine are essential for tissue repair and immune function [59]. Moreover, maintaining normoglycemia is key to preventing complications and promoting regeneration [62].

Another recognized relevant factor for healing is the absence of infection, as proper antimicrobial management reduces inflammation and facilitates granulation. Additionally, minimizing mechanical stress—particularly in pressure ulcers and diabetic foot ulcers—has been shown to significantly accelerate healing by preventing recurrent tissue trauma and supporting cellular regeneration [63].

Finally, patient adherence and education are pivotal. Consistent wound care practices and awareness of contributing behaviors (e.g., smoking cessation) improve outcomes [64].

4.1 Adherence to treatments

Adherence to treatment regimens is key in managing chronic wounds effectively, yet it remains challenging, as it requires complex strategies extending over long periods. Patients who consistently follow their prescribed plans are more likely to achieve successful healing faster.

A systematic review and meta-analysis comparing collagenase and papain-urea in wound debridement highlighted that while collagenase was effective, adherence to the treatment was critical for success [64].

Exploring factors influencing adherence, its prevalence and predictors, and as well as the effectiveness of supportive interventions is key to improving clinical outcomes in these patients.

High non-adherence rates to various therapies have been reported in patients with venous leg ulcers [65]. A systematic review found that non-adherence to compression therapy ranged from 2–42% in randomized controlled trials and 9.7–80% in real-world studies [66]. This review demonstrated that the median healing time of a venous ulcer is twice as long in poorly adherent patients. Patients and professionals' perspectives and motivations may differ, but as the interaction between patients and the healthcare team is pivotal in achieving concordance, a good understanding is necessary [66].

Factors influencing adherence include, firstly, comprehensible education provided by healthcare professionals on the importance of consistent treatment and proper self-care techniques. Low health literacy has been linked to non-adherence in diabetic ulcer treatment [67]. Secondly, the complexity of care regimens may involve frequent dressing changes, application of topical medications, and strict hygiene practices, which can be overwhelming, especially for older patients or those with cognitive impairments [68]. Thirdly, socioeconomic factors, since high costs of advanced care materials and treatments can be prohibitive for many patients, leading to skipped treatments or substitutions with less effective solutions [67]. Accessibility to specialized care services is another barrier, particularly in rural or underserved areas with limited resources. Finally, pain and psychological factors common in patients with chronic conditions, including depression and anxiety, are also critical [69].

The prevalence of non-adherence varies according to underlying diseases and treatment types. It has been hypothesized that non-adherence rates to treatment for venous ulcers range from 20–80%, while in pressure ulcers, rates can exceed 50% [65]. Predictors of non-adherence include comorbidities, wound severity, and lack of patient education on wound management [70].

Strategies to improve adherence should be multifaceted and tailored to individual needs. Educating patients and caregivers about wound management and the importance of adherence is fundamental. Clear instructions and demonstrations can improve treatment regimen execution. Incorporating patient feedback, allowing flexibility and effective pain management, is essential for improving comfort and willingness to engage in care [70].

Other strategies are focused on product preparations. Formulations that increase comfort are preferred, as those that minimize direct contact with the wound, also reducing infection occurrence. This is the case of pbserum SHS30®, useful to avoid infections and pain thanks to its single-dose microemulsion format. Future pbserum SHS30® integration into care protocols could transform the approach to chronic wound management.

Modulation of inflammation and fibrosis could also represent valuable approaches to facilitate healing. In this context, products containing hyaluronic acid such as pbserum HA1.5 High® exert anti-inflammatory and anti-fibrotic effects that can help limit these pathological processes, help to soften and reorganize dense scar tissue, thereby facilitating its progressive debridement and promote more effective healing [47, 48].

Optimizing these factors favoring healing often requires a multidisciplinary approach that combines clinical management with lifestyle interventions.

5. Limitations in chronic wound management

This chapter highlights current limitations in chronic wound management. Firstly, the increasing challenge of treating chronic wounds is closely tied to the global rise in chronic diseases, which complicates the management and the growing elderly population, as advanced age often exacerbates healing difficulties. This underscores the need to direct new efforts toward addressing the limitations associated with conventional treatments, such as infections, scarring, or further complications, which hinder wound management and negatively impact the patient's physical and psychological well-being [3]. Equally important is the effective management of pain. Another critical limitation is treatment adherence, a multifactorial issue that requires a multidisciplinary approach [67].

Ultimately, the development of innovative treatments capable of overcoming these barriers—offering economically accessible therapeutic options while simplifying wound care tasks—represents the "holy grail" in this field, paving the way for addressing the significant challenges currently faced.

6. Conclusions and future directions

Effective management of chronic wounds requires a tailored and often combined approach. No single method is ideal for all cases and healthcare providers must assess each wound individually to adjust treatment plans. The choice of treatment for chronic wounds should always be guided by wound characteristics, patient preferences, and overall goals of therapy.

For wound preparation, enzymatic debridement offers a balance between efficacy and preserving tissue integrity. This method is particularly effective for patients requiring a gentler approach or for wounds located in sensitive or cosmetically important areas where minimizing scarring is crucial. Concretely, collagenase presents a unique advantage due to its specificity and effectiveness in promoting a conducive healing environment and preserving tissue integrity. Further studies should continue exploring the use of collagenase in wound care, potentially leading to more effective and faster healing outcomes. Products tailored to enhance the enzymatic activity without the interference of additives that could compromise the healing environment or patient safety represent a significant advancement for chronic wounds.

Remarkably, while many treatments are available for chronic wounds, debridement is a key step that improves other therapies' effectiveness and contributes to the overall healing process, reducing scarring. Combining sharp surgical debridement with biologic or enzymatic techniques and complementing them with regenerative therapies (e.g., PRP, nanofat, and oxygen therapy) can maximize outcomes.

Recognizing barriers such as wound stalling, infection, and ischemia, and addressing them through personalized strategies, is essential for success. Moreover, adherence to treatments is crucial. Treatments and formulations promoting higher adherence rates and reducing pain and infections are preferable. Ongoing research and technological innovation will continue to refine the therapeutic landscape in wound management.

Acknowledgements

The authors would like to thank Rubén Lopez-Alalid and Javier Carrero from Premium Research, S.L., for their writing support.

Conflict of interest

The authors declare no conflict of interest.

Author details

Jorge Adrián Garza-Cerna[1], Gabriel Ángel Mecott-Rivera[1], Eugenia Paris Coronado[2], Yanko Castro-Govea[1], José Juan Pérez-Trujillo[3], Roberto Montes de Oca-Luna[3], Daniel Salas-Treviño[4], Guadalupe Tirma González-Mateo[5], Valeria Kopytina[6] and Jorge López Berroa[6]*

1 Plastic, Aesthetic and Reconstructive Surgery Service, University Hospital Dr. José Eleuterio González, Autonomous University of Nuevo León, Monterrey, Mexico

2 General Medicine and Physiotherapy, CIMA Hospital, San José, Costa Rica

3 Histology Department, Faculty of Medicine, Autonomous University of Nuevo León, Monterrey, Mexico

4 Infectious Diseases Service, University Hospital Dr. José Eleuterio González, Autonomous University of Nuevo León, Monterrey, Mexico

5 Premium Research, S.L., Guadalajara, Spain

6 Proteos Biotech Laboratories S.L., Madrid, Spain

*Address all correspondence to: jorge.lopez@proteosbiotech.com

References

[1] Falanga V, Isseroff RR, Soulika AM, Romanelli M, Margolis D, Kapp S, et al. Chronic wounds. Nature Reviews. Disease Primers. 2022;**8**(1):1-21

[2] Olsson M, Järbrink K, Divakar U, Bajpai R, Upton Z, Schmidtchen A, et al. The humanistic and economic burden of chronic wounds: A systematic review. Wound Repair and Regeneration. 2019;**27**(1):114-125

[3] Sen CK. Human wound and its burden: Updated 2020 compendium of estimates. Advances in Wound Care (New Rochelle). 2021;**10**(5):281-292

[4] Sen CK, Gordillo GM, Roy S, Kirsner R, Lambert L, Hunt TK, et al. Human skin wounds: A major and snowballing threat to public health and the economy. Wound Repair and Regeneration. 2009;**17**(6):763-771

[5] Mast BA, Diegelmann RF, Krummel TM, Cohen IK. Scarless wound healing in the mammalian fetus. Surgery, Gynecology & Obstetrics. 1992;**174**(5):441-451

[6] Hua Y, Bergers G. Tumors vs. chronic wounds: An immune cell's perspective. Frontiers in Immunology [Internet]. 2019;**10**. Available from: https://www.frontiersin.org/journals/immunology/articles/10.3389/fimmu.2019.02178/full

[7] Pastar I, Stojadinovic O, Yin NC, Ramirez H, Nusbaum AG, Sawaya A, et al. Epithelialization in wound healing: A comprehensive review. Advances in Wound Care. 2014;**3**(7):445-464

[8] Monika P, Chandraprabha MN, Rangarajan A, Waiker PV, Chidambara Murthy KN. Challenges in healing wound: Role of complementary and alternative medicine. Frontiers in Nutrition. 2022;**8**:791899

[9] Fonder MA, Lazarus GS, Cowan DA, Aronson-Cook B, Kohli AR, Mamelak AJ. Treating the chronic wound: A practical approach to the care of nonhealing wounds and wound care dressings. Journal of the American Academy of Dermatology. 2008;**58**(2):185-206

[10] Grey JE, Enoch S, Harding KG. Wound assessment. BMJ. 2006;**332**(7536):285-288

[11] Lindford AJ, Frey I, Vuola J, Koljonen V. Evolving practice of the Helsinki skin Bank. International Wound Journal. 2010;**7**(4):277-281

[12] Markiewicz-Gospodarek A, Kozioł M, Tobiasz M, Baj J, Radzikowska-Büchner E, Przekora A. Burn wound healing: Clinical complications, medical care, treatment, and dressing types: The current state of knowledge for clinical practice. International Journal of Environmental Research and Public Health. 2022;**19**(3):1338

[13] Falanga V, Saap LJ, Ozonoff A. Wound bed score and its correlation with healing of chronic wounds. Dermatologic Therapy. 2006;**19**(6):383-390

[14] Simms KW, Ennen K. Lower extremity ulcer management: Best practice algorithm. Journal of Clinical Nursing. 2011;**20**(1-2):86-93

[15] Nuutila K, Eriksson E. Moist wound healing with commonly available dressings. Advances in Wound Care (New Rochelle). 2021;**10**(12):685-698

[16] Yupanqui Mieles J, Vyas C, Aslan E, Humphreys G, Diver C, Bartolo P. Honey: An advanced antimicrobial and

wound healing biomaterial for tissue engineering applications. Pharmaceutics. 2022;**14**(8):1663

[17] Thomas DC, Tsu CL, Nain RA, Arsat N, Fun SS, Lah SN, et al. The role of debridement in wound bed preparation in chronic wound: A narrative review. Annals of Medicine and Surgery. 2021;**71**:102876

[18] Ramundo J, Gray M. Enzymatic wound debridement. Journal of Wound, Ostomy, and Continence Nursing. 2008;**35**(3):273-280

[19] Berwick D, Young L, Lee A, Lancaster D, Dheansa B. Local anaesthesia for enzymatic debridement of cutaneous burns: A prospective analysis of 27 cases. Annals of Burns and Fire Disasters. 2023;**36**(1):74-78

[20] Avila-Rodríguez MI, Meléndez-Martínez D, Licona-Cassani C, Manuel Aguilar-Yañez J, Benavides J, Lorena Sánchez M. Practical context of enzymatic treatment for wound healing: A secreted protease approach (Review). Biomedical Reports. 2020;**13**(1):3-14. DOI: 10.3892/br.2020.1300

[21] Nguyen HM, Ngoc Le TT, Nguyen AT, Thien Le HN, Pham TT. Biomedical materials for wound dressing: Recent advances and applications. RSC Advances. 2023;**13**(8):5509-5528

[22] Seswandhana MR, Kurniawan ID, Anwar SL, Humani HMA, Gabriela GC, Dachlan I, et al. The effects of negative pressure wound therapy on Vegf and angiogenesis in deep dermal burn injury: An experimental study. Annals of Burns and Fire Disasters. 2023;**36**(3):222-228

[23] Marra C, Pentangelo P, Losco L, Ceccaroni A, Barbato A, Alfano C. Lower extremity trauma: A multidimensional reconstructive approach with hyperbaric oxygen therapy. Journal of Clinical Medicine. 2024;**13**(5):1407

[24] Song H, Hao D, Zhou J, Farmer D, Wang A. Development of pro-angiogenic skin substitutes for wound healing. Wound Repair and Regeneration. 2024;**32**(3):208-216

[25] Chen B, Ke C, Zou S, et al. The therapeutic effect of concentrated growth factor gel on skin wounds with bone or tendon exposure. Journal of Wound Care. 2024;**33**(Sup2a):x-xiii. DOI: 10.12968/jowc.2024.33.Sup2a.x

[26] Alexander RW. Overview of use of Nanofat fully emulsified tSVF + HD platelet-rich plasma (PRP) in aesthetic and regenerative medicine cases. Medical Research Archives [S.l.]. Mar 2025;**13**(2). DOI: 10.18103/mra.v13i2.6260. ISSN 2375-1924. Available from: https://esmed.org/MRA/mra/article/view/6260 [Accessed: June 13, 2025]

[27] Harries RL, Bosanquet DC, Harding KG. Wound bed preparation: TIME for an update. International Wound Journal. 2016;**13**(S3):8-14

[28] Greco A, Mastronicola D, Pacini F, Giacomelli L, Papa S, Fiorentini C, et al. Researching the level of agreement among experts on terms used to describe wounds: An international study. International Wound Journal. 2023;**20**(8):2973-2980

[29] Choi E, Nahm FS, Han WK, Lee PB, Jo J. Topical agents: a thoughtful choice for multimodal analgesia. Korean Journal of Anesthesiology. 2020;**73**(5):384-393

[30] Steed DL. Debridement. The American Journal of Surgery. 2004;**187**(5):S71-S74

[31] Schultz GS, Sibbald RG, Falanga V, Ayello EA, Dowsett C, Harding K, et al. Wound bed preparation: a systematic

approach to wound management. Wound Repair and Regeneration. 2003;**11**(s1):S1-S28

[32] Molan PC. The evidence supporting the use of honey as a wound dressing. The International Journal of Lower Extremity Wounds. 2006;**5**(1):40-54

[33] Lam T, Beraja GE, Lev-Tov H. Efficacy of larval therapy for wounds: A systematic review and meta-analysis. Journal of Clinical Medicine. 2025;**14**(2):315

[34] Nowak M, Mehrholz D, Barańska-Rybak W, Nowicki RJ. Wound debridement products and techniques: Clinical examples and literature review. Postepy Dermatologii I Alergologii. 2022;**39**(3):479-490

[35] Hawthorne B, Simmons JK, Stuart B, Tung R, Zamierowski DS, Mellott AJ. Enhancing wound healing dressing development through interdisciplinary collaboration. Journal of Biomedical Materials Research. Part B, Applied Biomaterials. 2021;**109**(12):1967-1985

[36] Alvarez O, Fernandez-Obregon A, Rogers RS, Bergamo L, Masso J, Black M. A prospective, randomized, comparative study of collagenase and papain-urea for pressure ulcer debridement. Wounds. 2002;**14**(8):293-301

[37] Breite AG, McCarthy RC, Dwulet FE. Characterization and functional assessment of clostridium histolyticum class I (C1) collagenases and the synergistic degradation of native collagen in enzyme mixtures containing class II (C2) collagenase. Transplantation Proceedings. 2011;**43**(9):3171-3175

[38] Xue M, Le NT, Jackson CJ. Targeting matrix metalloproteases to improve cutaneous wound healing. Expert Opinion on Therapeutic Targets. 2006;**10**(1):143-155

[39] Marazzi M, Stefani A, Chiaratti A, Ordanini M, n., Falcone L, Rapisarda V. Effect of enzymatic debridement with collagenase on acute and chronic hard-to-heal wounds. Journal of Wound Care. 2006;**15**(5):222-227

[40] Saquib S, Carroll J, Flores C, Chestovich P. Management of pediatric pavement burns. Journal of Burn Care & Research. 2021;**42**(5):865-869

[41] Pham CH, Collier ZJ, Fang M, Howell A, Gillenwater TJ. The role of collagenase ointment in acute burns: a systematic review and meta-analysis. Journal of Wound Care. 2019;**28**(Sup2):S9-S15

[42] De Francesco F, De Francesco M, Riccio M. Hyaluronic acid/collagenase ointment in the treatment of chronic hard-to-heal wounds: An observational and retrospective study. Journal of Clinical Medicine. 2022;**11**(3):537

[43] Shu H, Xia Z, Qin X, Wang X, Lu W, Luo Q, et al. The clinical efficacy of collagen dressing on chronic wounds: A meta-analysis of 11 randomized controlled trials. Frontiers in Surgery. 2022;**9**:978407

[44] Fino P, Chello C, Latini C, Occhionorelli S, Moruzzi M, Scuderi N, et al. The combination of hyaluronic acid and collagenase in the treatment of skin ulcers: An open, multicenter clinical study assessing safety and tolerability of Bionect start®. European Review for Medical and Pharmacological Sciences. 2024;**28**(7):2894-2905

[45] Cakir M, Tekin A, Kucukkartallar T, Vatansev H, Kartal A. Enzymatic debridement in necrotizing pancreatitis. International Surgery. 2015;**100**(5):897-902

[46] Fronza M, Caetano GF, Leite MN, Bitencourt CS, Paula-Silva FWG, Andrade TAM, et al. Hyaluronidase modulates inflammatory response and accelerates the cutaneous wound healing. PLoS One. 2014;**9**(11):e112297

[47] Ruppert SM, Hawn TR, Arrigoni A, Wight TN, Bollyky PL. Tissue integrity signals communicated by high-molecular weight hyaluronan and the resolution of inflammation. Immunologic Research. 2014;**58**:186-192

[48] Petrey AC, de la Motte CA. Hyaluronan, a crucial regulator of inflammation. Frontiers in Immunology. 2014;**5**:101

[49] Sharp NE, Aguayo P, Marx DJ, Polak EE, Rash DE, Peter SD, et al. Nursing preference of topical silver sulfadiazine versus collagenase ointment for treatment of partial thickness burns in children: Survey follow-up of a prospective randomized trial. Journal of Trauma Nursing. 2014;**21**(5):253-257

[50] Hu D, Han Z, Li C, Lv L, Cheng Z, Liu S. Florfenicol induces more severe hemotoxicity and immunotoxicity than equal doses of chloramphenicol and thiamphenicol in Kunming mice. Immunopharmacology and Immunotoxicology. 2016;**38**(6):472-485

[51] Ferreira AM, Pereira Frota O, Rigotti MA, Alburquerque de Almeida W, da Silva Moura E, Christofoletti G. Topical therapy of wounds: Availability and use in primary health care centers. Journal of Nursing Ufpe Online [Internet]. 2015;**9**(Suppl.5):8401-8410. Available from: https://www.academia.edu/100380874/Topical_therapy_of_wounds_availability_and_use_in_primary_health_care_centers

[52] Greener B, Hughes A, Bannister NP, Douglass J. Proteases and pH in chronic wounds. Journal of Wound Care. 2005;**14**(2):59-61

[53] Sim P, Strudwick XL, Song Y, Cowin AJ, Garg S. Influence of acidic pH on wound healing in vivo: A novel perspective for wound treatment. International Journal of Molecular Sciences. 2022;**23**(21):13655

[54] Wilson MR, Nigam Y, Knight J, Pritchard DI. What is the optimal treatment time for larval therapy? A study on incubation time and tissue debridement by bagged maggots of the greenbottle fly, Lucilia sericata. International Wound Journal. 2019;**16**(1):219-225

[55] Manna B, Nahirniak P, Morrison CA. Wound Debridement. In: StatPearls [Internet]. Treasure Island (FL): StatPearls Publishing; 2025. Available from: http://www.ncbi.nlm.nih.gov/books/NBK507882/

[56] Mishra A, Kushare A, Gupta MN, Ambre P. Advanced dressings for chronic wound management. ACS Applied Bio Materials. 2024;**7**(5):2660-2676

[57] Horta-Velázquez A, Mota-Morales JD, Morales-Narváez E. Next-generation of smart dressings: Integrating multiplexed sensors and theranostic functions. International Journal of Biological Macromolecules. 2024;**254**(Pt 1):127737

[58] Study Details | Exciflex for Chronic Wound Therapy | ClinicalTrials.gov [Internet]. Available from: https://clinicaltrials.gov/study/NCT04887688?cond=Wound%20Healing&term=smart%20dressing&rank=3

[59] Guo S, DiPietro LA. Factors affecting wound healing. Journal of Dental Research. 2010;**89**(3):219

[60] Leenstra B, de Kleijn R, Kuppens G, Verhoeven BAN, Hinnen JW, de Borst GJ. Photo-optical transcutaneous oxygen tension measurement is of added value to predict diabetic foot ulcer healing: An observational study. Journal of Clinical Medicine. 2020;**9**(10):3291

[61] Wang SH, Shyu VBH, Chiu WK, Huang RW, Lai BR, Tsai CH. An overview of clinical examinations in the evaluation and assessment of arterial and venous insufficiency wounds. Diagnostics (Basel). 2023;**13**(15):2494

[62] Xiang J, Wang S, He Y, Xu L, Zhang S, Tang Z. Reasonable glycemic control would help wound healing during the treatment of diabetic foot ulcers. Diabetes Therapy. 2019;**10**(1):95-105

[63] Zhou S, Xie M, Su J, Cai B, Li J, Zhang K. New insights into balancing wound healing and scarless skin repair. Journal of Tissue Engineering. 2023;**14**:20417314231185848

[64] Patry J, Blanchette V. Enzymatic debridement with collagenase in wounds and ulcers: a systematic review and meta-analysis. International Wound Journal. 2017;**14**(6):1055-1065

[65] Van Hecke A, Grypdonck M, Defloor T. Interventions to enhance patient compliance with leg ulcer treatment: a review of the literature. Journal of Clinical Nursing. 2008;**17**(1):29-39

[66] Moffatt C, Kommala D, Dourdin N, Choe Y. Venous leg ulcers: Patient concordance with compression therapy and its impact on healing and prevention of recurrence. International Wound Journal. 2009;**6**(5):386-393

[67] Bouguettaya A, Gethin G, Probst S, Sixsmith J, Team V, Weller C. How health literacy relates to venous leg ulcer healing: A scoping review. PLoS One. 2023;**18**(1):e0279368

[68] Gould LJ, Abadir PM, White-Chu EF. Frailty, and impaired wound healing. In: Rosenthal RA, Zenilman ME, Katlic MR, editors. Principles and Practice of Geriatric Surgery [Internet]. Cham: Springer International Publishing; 2020. pp. 465-482. DOI: 10.1007/978-3-319-47771-8_27

[69] DiMatteo MR. Social support and patient adherence to medical treatment: a meta-analysis. Health Psychology. 2004;**23**(2):207-218

[70] Moffatt C, Murray S, Keeley V, Aubeeluck A. Non-adherence to treatment of chronic wounds: Patient versus professional perspectives. International Wound Journal. 2017;**14**(6):1305-1312

Chapter 3

Objective Clinical Approach to a Hard to Heal Wound of the Lower Limb in Diabetes

Juan Manuel Herrera-Arbelaez, Diego Morales-Suarez, Carolina Fonseca, Pascual Bernal-Ovalle and Daniel Santiago Cortés-Sarmiento

Abstract

The objective assessment by using measurement scales for hard-to-heal-wounds and patient's overall condition including associated pathologies should be the cornerstone in decision-making to enable the rational management of a lower extremity hard-to-heal-wound in a diabetic patient. Although the daily management of hard-to-heal-wounds in the community is usually performed by nursing services or the patient's family, medical coordination with the repeated evaluations of the wounds' status and the patient's general health is essential to achieve wound healing. The aim of the chapter is to explain in detail the step-by-step clinical evaluation and management of a hard-to-heal-wound using widely described tools that allow all stakeholders involved in the treatment, how to establish an objective common thread, based on clinical and paraclinical data, that should be well coordinated among physicians, nurses, and patient's family.

Keywords: hard-to-heal-wound, clinical assessment, wound assessment, tools decision-making, lower limb, diabetes

1. Introduction

Non-healing wounds are as old as humanity itself. In the animal kingdom, predators preferentially target weak or injured prey; thus, chronic wounds are virtually non-existent. Chronic wounds emerged in human history with the very consciousness of humanity, when human beings acquired awareness of their own existence, actions, and the external world. Human consciousness enabled us to learn, to learn to care, to create solutions for the care of other human beings, and to organize ourselves into care networks for those who were sick, weak, or injured. Consequently, a part of our very humanity is founded on the care of wounds suffered by others of our own species: Our humanity never allows us to abandon our weak or injured.

Throughout history, wound care has been a recurring theme in medical treatments. Before the advent of antibiotics, described treatments included cauterization with hot oil or incandescent metals, the use of procoagulant animal substances, local antiseptics, and ablative procedures such as amputation. For 250,000 years, humanity primarily dealt with acute wounds in a world with a life expectancy of less than 40 years. However, in the last 100 years, with the arrival of modern pharmacology (mainly antibiotic therapy) and the ability to treat chronic diseases like diabetes, we began to face wounds that were no longer acute but chronic. Now, our patients continue to live thanks to the treatment of their underlying condition; the wound may be free of infection due to antibiotic therapy, but the wound healing process stalls for various reasons, and the wound becomes a public health problem due to its chronicity.

Diabetes is a systemic disease characterized by elevated blood glucose levels (hyperglycemia), which in turn leads to a metabolic syndrome whose description is beyond the scope of this chapter. What is important to emphasize is that events such as sarcopenia, diabetic neuropathy, malnutrition, and obesity ultimately result in joint damage, deformities, and ulcers in the feet of diabetic patients. Often, given the systemic condition of the diabetic patient, ulcers or wounds become difficult-to-heal wounds due to systemic factors and the metabolic syndrome associated with diabetes. Additionally, there are also local wound factors that can lead to poor healing.

Hard-to-heal wounds represent a considerable financial burden for healthcare systems. Direct costs, such as hospitalizations, surgical interventions, and multiple therapies, often necessitated by complications, such as infection, osteomyelitis, or amputations, are high. Venous ulcers typically average £ 2200 pounds per year in the UK, while a hard-to-heal diabetic foot wound can cost up to four times as much (£ 8800 pounds). Wounds requiring ablative treatment through amputation reach £ 16,900 pounds. Outpatient nursing visits for dressings account for 62–78% of the total cost of treating a hard-to-heal wound. In addition, indirect costs (much more difficult to quantify) should be considered, including lost productivity, disability, and a deterioration in the patient's quality of life. The economic impact of these conditions is alarming. In the UK, the cost of treating diabetic ulcers to the National Health System (NHS) was estimated at £ 983 million in 2017/18, while the cost of treating venous ulcers for the same period was estimated at £ 1.3 billion (due to their higher frequency) [1, 2].

The objective of the chapter is to explain how all the systemic and local factors that hinder wound healing in the lower limbs of diabetic patients can be quantified, and with what tools, and how to resolve each particular situation.

The usual terminology of chronic or acute wound is no longer relevant in current practice. Currently, a wound that has not healed 40–50% of its surface area within a 4-week period is considered a difficult-to-heal wound, provided it has been managed with an appropriate standard of care. Under normal physiological conditions, a wound should heal more than 50% within 4 weeks. Because difficult-to-heal wounds commonly occur in patients with underlying health conditions such as diabetes, the guiding principle of wound management should be established on the definition and application of an appropriate standard of care (SoC).

An SoC has been defined as a series of actions that must be performed within a precise time frame during the wound treatment process [3]. This group of logical actions that define an appropriate SoC comprises the following 10 steps:

1. Holistic patient assessment: physical, psychological, spiritual, and social needs. This must include and identify the underlying pathophysiological cause(s) and risk factor(s)

2. Wound assessment: measurement

3. Decide the desired outcome (healing or maintenance) and care plan

4. Address/manage the underlying pathology or plan maintenance care

5. Implement local wound care according to WBP/TIME, etc., or maintenance/palliative care

6. Follow-up, reassessment, and measurement

7. Modify the care pathway and refer if necessary to specialists or Multi Disciplinary Team (MDT)

8. Patient/family education throughout the SoC

9. Discharge or transition for maintenance treatment to prevent recurrence

10. Record actions/outcomes at every episode of care.

In the case of difficult-to-heal wounds in diabetic patients, an appropriate SoC must objectify each action through the measurement of parameters that allow for rational treatment.

2. Holistic patient assessment

It is mostly related to patients' physical, psychological, spiritual, and social needs and certainly must include and identify the underlying pathophysiological cause(s) and risk factor(s) involved in the development of a hard to heal wound.

In diabetic patients, the disease itself defines both systemic risk factors and local wound factors. The first thing to consider is that if the disease can be managed on an outpatient basis, the ulcer or wound can be as well, and that is why establishing the appropriate standard of care is so important. **Table 1** shows the general treatment goals for the diabetic patient (systemic).

2.1 Systemic factors

Excess weight should be reduced by 5–10% per year, and the patient should generally be below 130% of their ideal Body Mass Index (BMI) [4]. While excess weight alone is not a risk factor for ulcers, an overweight diabetic patient is at risk of developing metabolic syndrome, in which the risk of developing neuropathy due to diabetes increases, as do their glycated hemoglobin levels, blood pressure values, low-density lipoprotein cholesterol, and triglyceride levels. It is also highly associated with a reduction in physical activity, which in turn reduces proprioception and leads to sarcopenia in those over 45 years of age. It is absolutely mandatory to weigh the patient at each wound check and monitor their weight.

Glycated hemoglobin (HbA1c) serves as a marker of glycemic control throughout the day. Elevated HbA1c levels correlate with an increased risk of diabetic neuropathy, a significant contributing factor to recalcitrant lower extremity wounds. Rapid

Tests	Follow-up	Target
Weight	Regularly or as indicated	Weight <130% of ideal body weight or BMI <27
Hemoglobin A1c	Every 6 months, or every 3 if above target	Less than 8% (ideal <7%)
Lipid screening (LDL cholesterol)	Annually	Less than 100 mg/dL
Microalbuminuria	Annually	Negative or less than 30 mg/24 h
Serum creatinine	Annually	0.6–1.2 mg/dL
Albumin/globulin ratio	Annually	Albumin: 3.5–5.0 g/dLGlobulins: 2.0–3.5 g/dLRatio: 1.1–2.5
Blood pressure	Every visit	Systolic <130 / Diastolic <85
Visual foot exam	Every visit	Good skin integrity; correction and protection of foot deformities
Monofilament testing	Annually	Sensitivity with Semmes-Weinstein 5.07 (10g) monofilament
Skin and musculoskeletal exam	Every visit	Good skin integrity; correction and protection of musculoskeletal issues
Dilated pupil retinal exam	Annually	Stabilization or no progression of retinopathy
Smoking status	Annually or as indicated	No tobacco use
Modified Romberg test	Annually or as indicated	>20 seconds; minimum tolerated: 11 seconds

Table 1.
Reference values in diabetes.

correction of HbA1c values with insulin therapy can also induce iatrogenic neuropathy, known as treatment-induced neuropathy of diabetes (TIND), characterized by the acute onset of neuropathic pain and/or autonomic dysfunction within 8 weeks following a substantial improvement in glycemic control, typically defined as a decrease in HbA1c of ≥2 percentage points over 3 months [5–7]. Iron deficiency complicates HbA1c control, potentially necessitating more aggressive insulin regimens. Furthermore, red blood cell turnover in the bone marrow, along with erythrocyte quality and heterogeneity, can influence the rate of hemoglobin glycation. Iron deficiency, by altering hemoglobin structure and inducing peroxidation, accelerates this glycation process, which is relevant in the context of anemia due to iron deficiency. Consequently, inadequate HbA1c control signifies suboptimal disease management and, therefore, diminished capacity for wound healing in the patient.

The assessment of hyperlipidemia is performed within the context of the established relationship where the pathogenic factors of hyperglycemia, hyperlipidemia, adipokines, and insulin resistance induce oxidative stress in endothelial cells in the setting of diabetes [8]. While nerves are more susceptible to the reduced vascularity and oxygen availability resulting from diabetic microangiopathy, all tissues, including the skin, are also affected. Locally, diabetic microangiopathy not only impairs oxygen availability in the wound but also alters the pH within the wound bed.

Microalbuminuria is a marker of diabetic nephropathy, which is secondary to neuropathy; it is usually the earliest of the indirect markers of diabetic neuropathy and metabolic syndrome. Microalbuminuria is closely associated with the presence of arterial hypertension (in 70% of patients) and also with the presence of tumor necrosis factor α (TNF-α) in urine, indicative of systemic chronic inflammatory processes. Locally, this interplay of systemic alterations affects both the temperature at the wound site and the pH of the wound bed [9, 10].

Serum creatinine is also a marker of renal function, associated with nephropathy when its levels increase. However, in older diabetic patients with otherwise normal renal function, a decreased serum creatinine level can sometimes go unnoticed, which may be related to severe sarcopenia or chronic malnutrition.

The albumin/globulin ratio allows for a rapid assessment of the patient's overall nutritional status. Its value should be evaluated within the context of malnutrition, which can be determined using the Mini Nutritional Assessment-Short Form (MNA-SF), and sarcopenia, which can be assessed using SARC-F and handgrip strength [11, 12]. It is important to remember that hypoalbuminemia is often associated with transudation through intact skin, and in the case of difficult-to-heal wounds, a subtle transudate can be mistaken for wound exudate. Additionally, hypoalbuminemia-induced changes in osmotic pressure lead to edema and fluid retention, causing weight gain in the patient even when they are actually malnourished.

The periodic evaluation of foot skin sensitivity with Semmes-Weinstein 5.07 monofilaments (10 gr) is an indirect marker of diabetic neuropathy.

The other readily accessible clinical site for neuropathy assessment is through the annual retinal examination that diabetic patients should undergo [13].

Within the holistic evaluation, it is crucial never to overlook questions about smoking, which has been extensively linked to impaired wound healing.

The proprioception examination of the foot should be performed using the Herrera test (modified Romberg). A lower limb lacking proprioception will present with difficult-to-heal wounds, especially plantar foot ulcers, because the patient does not sense pressure, lacks an unconscious perception of the limb's position in space, and usually does not feel vibration either. Without these proprioceptive sensations (pressure, position, and vibration), the patient has lost all defense mechanisms against repetitive microtrauma that normally function in healthy individuals. Since these sensations are unconscious, the patient does not report having lost them or having them diminished, and therefore, they must be routinely evaluated by healthcare professionals.

3. Wound assessment: Measurement

As defined by the TIMERS consensus, parameters that should be assessed include depth, volume, extent, area, exudate (amount and type), location, appearance, temperature, odor, overt and subclinical infection, and structural deformity. However, classifications have been traditionally used to determine the type of chronic wound in the diabetic patient, its prognosis, and the management plan to follow. The rationale for using classifications stems from the significant impact of lower extremity wounds in diabetic individuals. Furthermore, the cost of managing lower extremity wounds in diabetics places a substantial burden on healthcare system financing annually worldwide [14].

Difficult-to-heal wounds can affect up to a quarter of individuals with diabetes during their lifetime, with a global annual incidence of 6.3%, and an estimated prevalence reaching up to 25% of diabetic patients, with the higher rates in men than in women. Difficult-to-heal diabetic foot wounds impose a significant individual disease burden; once they occur, they increase mortality in diabetic patients by 2.5 times in the following 5 years compared to those without lower extremity wounds. Difficult-to-heal wounds in diabetics are also the most common cause of non-traumatic amputations worldwide. Worldwide, the prevalence of so-called diabetic foot (including hard-to-heal wounds) among patients with diabetes mellitus is 8–13%, mainly affecting patients aged between 45 and 65. The amputation risk is up to 15 times higher in patients with diabetes than in patients without diabetes. Amputation incidence in patients with diabetes is around 2.5–6 per 1000 patients per year [15].

One of the most serious complications of type 2 diabetes mellitus is the presence of difficult-to-heal inframalleolar wounds, which has been termed "diabetic foot" in the literature. This concept encompasses a range of physiological alterations such as peripheral neuropathy, immune system deficiencies, and micro- and macrovascular disease [16, 17].

Lower extremity wounds in diabetic patients necessitate the evaluation not only of the wound itself but also its systemic and local causes, which can be summarized as biological and mechanical. Accordingly, multiple classifications have been proposed for difficult-to-heal lower extremity wounds in diabetic individuals.

3.1 Wagner classification

The most well-known and widely used classification globally assesses vascular involvement, neuropathy, and the status of necrosis or gangrene, categorizing them into five grades based on their severity according to their characteristics, with Grade I being the least severe and Grade V defining extensive gangrene with the characteristics of involvement of the entire foot (see **Table 2**).

3.1.1 University of Texas classification

This classification, like the previous one, is popularized for its ease of application. Developed at the University of Texas Health Science Center at San Antonio by Lavery and Armstrong in 1996 and validated in 1998, its main characteristic is that it assesses the diabetic foot in 4 grades, from 0 to 4, and dimensions the damage or lesion with severity parameters of infection and ischemia, and the combination of both (see **Table 3**).

3.1.2 PEDIS classification

This is a classification that involves the evaluation of variables, by their acronym in English, depth, infection, and sensation, and was created to support research groups with the aim of suggesting a classification that is universally understood. It was

Grade	Injury	Characteristics
0	None	Hyperkeratosis, Prominence of metatarsal heads, Claw toes, Bony deformities
I	Superficial ulcers	full-thickness, skin destruction
II	Deep ulcers	Penetrates skin, fat, and ligaments without bone involvement
III	Deep ulcer with abscess (osteomyelitis)	extensive and deep, with discharge and malodor (Bad smell)
IV	Limited gangrene	Distal foot necrosis
V	Extensive gangrene	Entire foot involvement

Table 2.
Wagner classification.

Stages	**Grade**			
	0	**I**	**II**	**III**
A	Pre- or post-ulcerative site that has healed (epithelialized)	Superficial wound not involving tendon, capsule, or bone	Wound penetrating to tendon or capsule.	Wound penetrating bone or joint.
B	Nonischemic, infected wounds.	Nonischemic, infected wounds.	Nonischemic, infected wounds.	Nonischemic, infected wounds.
C	Ischemic, non-infected wounds.	Ischemic, non-infected wounds.	Ischemic, non-infected wounds.	Ischemic, non-infected wounds.
D	Ischemic and infected wounds (both present)	Ischemic and infected wounds (both present)	Ischemic and infected wounds (both present)	Ischemic and infected wounds (both present)

Table 3.
University of Texas classification.

created by the "International Working Group on the Diabetic Foot (IWGDF) in 2003 [18, 19]."

Many other classifications exist that base their evaluation and validation criteria on lesion criteria of the skin, degree of infection, and depth, such as the Gibbons classification, or others that categorize gangrene by degrees of increasing to decreasing complexity, like the less well-known Pecoraro classification. These generally focus on describing factors associated with the wound and do not include the aggravating factors that lead to the acute diabetic foot attack.

3.1.3 Saint Elian classification (also referred as Saint Elian)

The Latin American Saint Elian classification system for diabetic foot is an objective scale that includes 10 evaluation factors, each assigned a score of 1 to 3 according to its degree of severity. It provides information about the severity based on factors such as location, topography, and the number of affected areas, and categorizes the patient into a severity grade (minor to major) derived from the presence of aggravating factors, such as: ischemia, infection, edema, and neuropathy. It is complemented by three local and characteristic wound factors including area, depth, and healing phase.

Upon establishing the patient's conditions and including them in this classification, the scores obtained for each factor are summed, resulting in a severity score categorized as mild I (less than 10 points), moderate II (11–20 points), and severe III (21–30 points). According to the grade obtained for the patient, the prognosis of each lesion is defined, and the most appropriate treatment is established. The Saint Elián system mandates periodic re-evaluation or re-grading, allowing for the observation of changes in the patient and their wound over time, thereby enabling the simultaneous tracking of patient and lesion evolution.

Although the classification predates current consensus guidelines, it is the only classification system for difficult-to-heal wounds that aligns with the modern wound management principles such as the TIMERS consensus, hence the increasing preference for its use in diabetic patients.

Reasons for using the Saint Elian classification:

1. For reclassifying DM foot injuries

2. For visualizing improvements in the clinical conditions of grades II and III

3. For reassessing wounds to visualize improvement in healing

4. For gaining information regarding failed procedures that may lead to amputation/death

5. For analyzing the patient in a comprehensive and not so specific way (considering that the foot is a part of the body).

4. Deciding the desired outcome (healing or maintenance) and care plan

In the case of diabetic patients, deciding the desired outcome (healing or maintenance) and the care plan depends largely on the scores obtained in the Saint Elian classification (See **Tables 4** and **5**) and the patient's overall condition, as well as the setting in which the decision is made (inpatient/outpatient). In patients with terminal processes due to associated pathologies, the decision will always be based on the concept of alleviating or palliating the disease.

5. Addressing/managing the underlying pathology or plan maintenance care

5.1 Effect of diabetes on wound healing

The physiology of wound healing depends on the interaction of various cell lines, divided into four distinct stages: hemostasis, inflammation, proliferation, and remodeling [17]. This sequential process is negatively altered in patients with diabetes mellitus due to the effect of hyperglycemia, which leads to an increased production of advanced glycation end products (AGEs), thereby disrupting the formation of the extracellular matrix (ECM), the cellular migration of polymorphonuclear leukocytes (PMNs) (diapedesis), and the release of pro-inflammatory cytokines such as vascular endothelial growth factor (VEGF) and transforming growth factor β (TGF-β) [20].

Saint Elian score system					
Factors		**Score (severity)**			
		1 point (Mild)	**2 points (Moderate)**	**3 points (severe)**	**Score**
Anatomical	1. Primary zone (location)	Phalanges	Metatarsal	Tarsal	
	2. Topographic aspects (location)	Dorsal or plantar	Lateral or medial	Two or more	
	3. Zone number	One	Two	Three (multiple wounds)	

Saint Elian score system					
Factors		**Score (severity)**			
		1 point (Mild)	**2 points (Moderate)**	**3 points (severe)**	**Score**
Aggravating factors	4. Ischemia	Palpable pulses slightly diminished ABI (0.89-0.70) TBI (0.74-0.60)	Scarcely palpable pulses	Non palpable pulses	
			ABI (0.89-0.70	ABI (< 0.50)	
			TBI (0.74-0.60)	TBI (< 0.30)	
	5. Infection	Erythema < 2 cm. Purulent discharge, warmth, tenderness	Erythema > 2 cm. Muscles, tendons, or bone or joint infection	Systemic inflammatory response Syndrome. Secondary hyper or hypoglycemia	
	6. Edema	Periwound	One foot or leg	Bilateral secondary to comorbidities	
	7. Neuropathy	Protective Sensation diminished (128 Hz Tuning fork, Semmes-Weinstein, vibratip, Ipswich)	Protective Sensation absent (128 Hz Tuning fork, Semmes-Weinstein, vibratip, Ipswich)	Diabetic neuroosteoarthropathy (DNOA) - Charcot arthropathy	
Tissue involvement	8. Area	Small < 10 cm^2	Medium 11-40 cm^2	Big > 40 cm^2	
	9. Depth	Superficial (skin)	Tendons, fascia, muscles	Deep joint and bones	
	10. Wound healing phase	Inflammatory	Granulating	Epithelialization	

For aggravating factors a 0 (None) score can be obtained. ABI Ankle Brachial Index, sometimes also referred as ABPI Ankle Brachial Pressure Index.

Table 4.
Saint Elian score system.

Score sum		
Final score	**Grade (Severity)**	**Prognosis**
< 10	I (Mild)	Likely successful wound healing. No LEA
11-20	II (Moderate)	Partial foot threatening: outcome related to "state-of-the-art" therapies used and associated with a good patient biological response. <30% LEA.
21-30	III (Severe)	Limb and life threatening: outcome unrelated to "state-of-the-art" therapies used because of poor biological patient response. < 30% LEA.

LEA Lower extremity amputation.

Table 5.
Grade and prognosis of Saint Elian Score System.

In diabetic individuals, the first phase of healing (inflammatory) is prolonged because the function of polymorphonuclear leukocytes is negatively affected, and their response to exogenous bacterial microorganisms is diminished, thus allowing bacterial colonization and subsequent wound infection, which culminates in the chronicity of the wounds [21].

Subsequently, in the second phase of healing, the proliferative phase—which occurs after the first week of the initial injury—fibroblasts, the most active cells during this period, decrease their production of extracellular matrix and collagen. Concurrently, keratinocytes cannot migrate adequately from the wound edges toward the center due to a local fibrosis process that hinders the action of myofibroblasts, limiting wound closure. Finally, there is also endothelial dysfunction due to the microvascular pathology in diabetic patients, which generates tissue hypoxia, a decrease in the availability of local nitric oxide, and consequently leads to reduced angiogenesis and tissue ischemia, depriving the affected soft tissues of optimal oxygenation and therefore the capacity for regeneration [22].

5.2 Diabetic complications that affect wound healing

All the factors mentioned above keep wounds in people with diabetes in a constant state of inflammation, especially in areas like the lower limbs where there is less oxygen compared to healthy individuals. This ongoing inflammation makes it harder for the skin to grow, causing it to become chronic, even when proper treatment is given.

5.3 Peripheral neuropathy

Peripheral neuropathy is one of the most important risk factors for developing hard-to-heal wounds in patients with diabetes mellitus. This condition is present in half of all people with diabetes and the most sensitive test to diagnose it is the monofilament test, as previously described [23, 24].

5.4 Peripheral neuropathy subtypes

Peripheral neuropathy can be classified into motor, sensory, and autonomic types. Motor neuropathy causes atrophy of the intrinsic muscles of the foot, which leads to foot deformities and the development of pressure points. These pressure areas increase the risk of hard-to-heal wounds due to repetitive microtrauma.

Sensory neuropathy results in the loss of protective sensation, as previously described. Finally, autonomic neuropathy causes dry skin and loss of skin. This leads to impaired wound healing (because hair follicles are the major sites of keratinocyte activity) and increases the risk of skin infections [25, 26].

Several clinical tests can help diagnose diabetic neuropathy. The monofilament test (see Image 1) is a useful screening tool with a sensitivity and specificity greater than 80% for detecting sensory loss in the feet [27].

In comparison, the Ipswich Touch Test evaluates light touch sensation and has been shown to have a sensitivity of 51–83% and specificity of 96–98% when compared to the monofilament test. Meanwhile, the 128 Hz tuning fork vibration test has demonstrated better sensitivity (76–100%) and specificity (90–96%) for detecting sensory neuropathy [28].

5.5 Proprioceptive testing: Herrera test

Herrera proprioceptive test (also known as the modified Romberg test) is the only physical exam tool available to assess proprioception. A normal test result ranges from 20 to 40 seconds, and the minimum protective threshold to prevent joint injuries in the foot is 12 seconds.

When proprioception is lost, not only is the skin's natural protection, but Charcot arthropathy may also take place, leading to foot deformities. Since deformities can cause wounds, evaluating a patient's proprioceptive status is essential.

Although the traditional approach for non-healing foot wounds is to offload the foot using walkers or total contact casts, this can further decrease proprioception due to the lack of sensory input. As a result, this practice is being increasingly reconsidered, especially now that there is an objective tool available to assess the proprioceptive function [29].

5.6 Advanced evaluation of peripheral nervous function and imaging findings

Similarly, for a more detailed assessment of peripheral nerve function, there are complementary diagnostic tools such as nerve conduction studies and electromyography (EMG), which provide an objective understanding of axonal injury. These tests help differentiate diabetic neuropathy from other peripheral neuropathies. When compared to the clinical tests described earlier, nerve conduction studies and EMG show a sensitivity of 94% and specificity of 62%.

In terms of imaging, plain radiographs are useful for identifying morphological changes in the typical radiographic anatomy of the foot. In patients with Charcot neuroarthropathy, findings may include joint subluxation, bone fragmentation, collapse of the plantar arch, and loss of calcaneal pitch. These features are particularly important because they are associated with a higher risk of pressure zones and resulting ulcerations in the lower limbs, especially in the advanced stages of the disease [30].

Regarding future prospects, emerging technologies for the study of peripheral neuropathy include retinal studies such as visual evoked potentials and electroretinography, which show promise for detecting early subclinical retinal dysfunction. However, despite their potential, these technologies currently have limited routine clinical use [31–33].

5.7 Peripheral arterial disease

Peripheral arterial disease (PAD) occurs secondary to atherosclerosis and is a major macrovascular and microvascular complication in patients with diabetes. It typically affects infrapopliteal vessels [34].

PAD leads to reduced oxygen and nutrient delivery to tissues distal to the vascular obstruction, resulting in chronic limb ischemia and negatively impacting tissue regeneration. This increases the risk of infection, gangrene, and ultimately amputation [35, 36]. Evaluation is performed through arterial Doppler and/or angiography. Angiography is essential to map the possible vascular bridges between foot angiosomes.

The foot has a natural protective mechanism present from birth: Collapsed arterioles exist between different angiosomes. Due to pressure gradients, these vessels can become permeable by the third week after circulatory collapse in an angiosome, allowing neighboring angiosomes to supply the affected area. This is one of the reasons why foot wounds generally have a longer exudative phase (up to 21 days) compared to wounds in other parts of the body.

5.8 Immune dysfunction

The immune system in people with diabetes mellitus is impaired through multifactorial mechanisms. Chronic inflammation affects polymorphonuclear function and disrupts cell signaling [37].

In general, diabetic macrophages are hyperreactive, releasing pro-inflammatory cytokines even in response to minor stimuli, thereby perpetuating local inflammation. However, compared to non-diabetics, these cells have a reduced ability to phagocytose microorganisms, which promotes wound infection and the development of biofilm, often seen in diabetic foot ulcers [38, 39].

Many diabetic patients—especially older adults—also suffer from protein-calorie malnutrition, often accompanied by deficiencies in vitamins A, C, and D, and low serum levels of electrolytes such as magnesium, zinc, and iron. These deficiencies impair extracellular collagen production, reduce immune response due to low antibody and immune protein production, and lead to poor angiogenesis [40, 41].

Diabetic patients frequently have other comorbidities, such as chronic kidney disease, heart failure, and obesity, which further impair healing. Specifically:

- Chronic kidney disease increases uremic toxins, inhibiting cell proliferation and angiogenesis.

- Congestive heart failure leads to persistent tissue hypoxia due to reduced cardiac output.

- Obesity creates a low-grade inflammatory state that adds to that caused by hyperglycemia and increases mechanical pressure on the lower limbs, raising the risk of soft tissue injuries.

6. Implement local wound care according to TIMERS or maintenance/palliative care

Each wound is unique due to the wide variety of influencing factors. Therefore, it is essential to recognize common patterns across different wounds. For this purpose, conceptual frameworks have been developed to manage chronic wounds. The most current and recommended is the TIMERS framework (see **Table 6**).

TIMERS is a revised version of the traditional TIME framework, which has been valuable for chronic wound management. It includes two additional components:

- R for Repair

- S for Social factors

Since chronic wounds are primarily managed on an outpatient basis, the patient's social context plays a vital role in healing.

TIMERS is a methodology in which, based on clinical observation, the wound type is classified, and a treatment option is selected that matches the findings, all aimed at achieving a predefined healing outcome.

TIMERS framework for managing hard-to-heal wounds in diabetic foot.				
Treat underlying cause and risk factors				
T: Tissue	**I: Inflammation/ Infection**	**M: Moisture**	**E: Edge**	**R: Repair**
Observation: devitalized tissue	Observation: inflammation and/or infection, bioburden	Observation: incorrect moisture balance	Observation: edge rolled/epibole/ callus. Poor advancement of wound edge	Observation: Slow/stalled closure failing conservative therapy
Debridment options: Autolytic, sharp surgical, mechanical including; debridement pads, enzymatic (collagenase, lipase, liase preparations)	Treatment options: Antimicrobials Antibiotics Biofilm pathway Bacterial binding dressings, enzymatic (collagenase, lipase, liase preparations), platelet-rich plasma (PRP) as local antibiotic delivery system (R).	Treatment options: NPWT Compression Absorbent dressings	Treatment options: See also debridement Excision of sclerosed margins Wound fillers (e.g., collagen, hyaluronic Acid)	Treatment options: Cell scaffold ECM-based technologies Growth factors Platelet-rich plasma (PRP), Bioengineered substitutes, Stem cell therapy, Autologous skin graft
Outcome: Clean wound bed, debride devitalized tissue	Outcome: Inflammation, infection and biofilm controlled	Outcome: Manage moisture Wound environment conducive to healing	Outcome: Reduced wound size Epithelialization	Outcome: Wound closure, repair tissue
S: Social- and patient-related factors				
Social situation Patient understanding Patient adherence Patient choice Psychosocial	→	Engage the patient with the care plan	→	Patient education Understanding belief system Motivational literacy Active listening Psychoeducation Patient's own goals. Patient's family/ caregiver education
Epidermal and other growth factors were not included because there is a debate on systemic effects about them.				

Table 6.
TIMERS framework for managing hard-to-heal wounds in diabetic foot.

6.1 Treatment of diabetic foot ulcers

Principles of treatment:

- Debridement: Essential for removing necrotic tissue, debris, and bacterial biofilm. It can be performed using surgical, enzymatic, autolytic, or mechanical techniques, depending on the wound type and available resources.

- Infection control: The presence of infection must be evaluated both clinically and microbiologically. Mild infections may respond to oral antibiotics and local care, while moderate-to-severe infections often require hospitalization, intravenous antibiotics, and sometimes urgent surgical intervention.

- Exudate management and dressings: The choice of dressing should be guided by the amount of exudate, the condition of the wound bed, and the presence or absence of infection. Modern dressings such as hydrocolloids, hydrogels, foams, alginates, silver-based dressings, or collagenase help maintain an optimal moist environment for healing.

- Off-loading: One of the most effective strategies in managing plantar ulcers is pressure redistribution using off-loading devices. Options include removable braces, therapeutic footwear, or custom insoles.

- Metabolic control: Proper glycemic control is essential. Hyperglycemia promotes chronic inflammation, immune dysfunction, and delayed wound healing.

- Advanced therapies: In complex or slow-healing cases, advanced therapies may be considered, including negative pressure wound therapy, growth factors, mesenchymal stem cellular therapies, and hyperbaric oxygen therapy.

6.2 Mesenchymal stem cells

Mesenchymal stem cells (MSCs) are multipotent stromal cells that can be isolated from various tissues, including bone marrow, adipose tissue, and umbilical cord blood. Among these, umbilical cord-derived MSCs have gained significant attention due to their non-invasive collection, high proliferation capacity, and immunomodulatory properties. In foot and ankle surgery, MSC-based therapies have shown promise in enhancing tissue regeneration, reducing inflammation, and promoting healing in conditions such as chronic ulcers, tendon injuries, and post-surgical wound complications. These cells exert their therapeutic effects not only through differentiation but also *via* paracrine signaling, notably through the secretion of exosomes—nano-sized vesicles rich in proteins, lipids, and RNA that modulate the local microenvironment and stimulate repair [42].

A prominent example of research in the field of diabetes is the study titled "Umbilical Cord-Derived Mesenchymal Stem Cell-Derived Exosomes Combined Pluronic F127 Hydrogel Promote Chronic Diabetic Wound Healing and Complete Skin Regeneration." This work explores a novel therapeutic strategy for the complex chronic wounds that affect diabetic patients, for which there are still no fully effective treatments.

The main objective of the researchers was to evaluate whether a combination of exosomes derived from human umbilical cord mesenchymal stem cells (hUCMSC-exos) and a Pluronic F-127 hydrogel (PF-127) could enhance wound healing. To this end, they topically applied hUCMSC-exos encapsulated in a thermosensitive PF-127 hydrogel to full-thickness skin wounds in a streptozotocin-induced diabetic rat model. The results revealed a significant improvement in granulation tissue regeneration and a positive regulation in the expression of key factors involved in wound healing, such as vascular endothelial growth factor (VEGF) and transforming growth factor beta-1 (TGFB-1). In conclusion, this combined therapy, based on biomaterials and exosomes, emerges as a promising therapeutic approach for skin regeneration in chronic diabetic wounds [43].

6.3 Other biomaterials

Biomaterials constitute a field of research characterized by constant innovation. For the application of biomaterials, hard-to-heal wounds can be classified into two types: tunneled wounds and non-tunneled wounds. Accordingly, there are two primary types of biomaterials: those primarily used for wounds involving only soft tissue and those used for tunneled wounds.

In the foot, a tunneled wound always necessitates surgical debridement. Due to the shallow soft tissues of the foot, these types of wounds are generally associated with bone infection (osteomyelitis). For superficial wounds, common biomaterials treatments include hydrocolloids, hydrogels, injectable nanocomposites, foams, needleless electrospinning technology, films, membranes, polymers, and, most recently, silk fibroin nanofibers, as detailed in **Table 6** according to TIMERS.

For tunneled wounds, the use of bone substitutes preloaded with antibiotics (tobramycin and gentamicin), platelet-rich plasma (PRP) preloaded with antibiotics (which can be used according to antibiogram results), or osteoconductive S53P4 bioactive glass (composed of silicon dioxide, calcium oxide, phosphorus pentoxide, and sodium oxide) has gained increasing relevance. S53P4 increases the local pH in the tunneled wound, inhibiting bacterial colonization while simultaneously generating osteoinduction by locally converting calcium and phosphate to hydroxyapatite [44–46]. Generally, the use of PRP preloaded with antibiotics and S53P4 bioactive glass in tunneled wounds is preferred, either combined or individually, depending on the surgical assessment of the tunneling depth [47, 48].

6.4 Patient adherence and psychological factors

Optimal treatment of chronic diseases requires strong patient adherence to medical management, and diabetes and its complications are no exception.

However, intrinsic behavioral and mental health factors in diabetic patients can negatively affect self-care. For example, depression is associated with poor glycemic control and thus delayed wound healing. Similarly, cognitive impairment, which is common in elderly diabetics—affecting up to 50% of this population—interferes with adherence to non-pharmacological wound care strategies [48].

Similarly, chronic psychological stress impacts wound healing by increasing systemic cortisol production leads to immunosuppression (allowing bacterial colonization and infection of wounds) and also reduces the synthesis of collagen in the extracellular matrix.

Last but not least, the psychosocial context also plays a fundamental role in the pathophysiology of hard-to-heal wounds. In general, social determinants of health—such as low socioeconomic status, limited access to the healthcare system, and geographical barriers in the case of individuals living in rural areas—hinder optimal and timely intervention for diabetic patients and are associated with the worse clinical outcomes.

7. Follow-up, reassessment, and measurement

Although primary wound management is usually carried out by specialized wound care centers or by the patient's family, the most important aspect is recognizing when a wound is not responding to initial treatment. This is the same criterion used to define a hard-to-heal wound.

In cases where the healing response is less than 40–50% after 4 weeks, it is appropriate to consider underlying causes that may not be evident during routine clinical evaluation, including the possibility of a neoplasm. Appropriate diagnostic tests such as biopsy and histological analysis should be considered, and the patient should be referred accordingly.

In chronic wounds, which show prolonged progression with a halt in the inflammatory phase, it is essential to assess the presence of biofilm, persistent necrotic tissue, local hypoxia, pH changes, and signs of critical colonization.

7.1 Enzymatic management

When a skin wound occurs, a series of events aimed at repairing the skin lesion are instantly initiated and are usually divided into three overlapping phases:

- Inflammatory phase.
- Proliferative phase: tissue granulation, epithelialization and angiogenesis.
- Extracellular matrix remodeling phase.

In the inflammatory phase, leukocytes invade the injured tissue and begin to clear debris, both dead tissue and contaminants and bacteria. Platelets and inflammatory cells then release mediators to trigger the further healing process. Therefore, modern therapies tend to combine recombinant enzymes (collagenase, lyase, and lipase) with hyaluronic acid [49].

Collagenases are a very versatile group of molecules due to the large number of processes in which they are involved in the organism and the new applications that have been described for their therapeutic use. They are enzymes that have the ability to break collagen peptide bonds at physiological pH. They belong to the family of matrix metalloproteinases; they are involved in physiological processes on which the integrity of collagen or its rearrangement depends.

It should be remembered that collagen is the most abundant fibrillar protein in the human body and collagenases are indispensable for its proper functioning, for example, during collagen synthesis, procollagen must first be fragmented by a collagenase in order to be "reassembled" into mature fibers [50].

In medicine, collagenases are used to treat burns and ulcers, remove scar tissue and in organ transplantation. They are normally involved in the repair process of the dermis and also assist in the granulation and re-epithelialization stage.

Collagenase is an exogenous enzyme that breaks down native and denatured collagen. However, collagenase will not degrade normal, healthy collagen. Collagenase and other debridement enzymes may play an important role in the healing process by facilitating the removal of necrotic tissue and promoting the formation of healthy granulation tissue according to some authors [51].

Modern recombinant collagenase do not contain any antibiotic in their composition to treat possible complications due to infection (they do not present the potential problems associated with chloramphenicol), but the presence in their formulation of another enzyme such as r-lyase helps to reduce the viscosity of biological fluids, increasing vascular permeability and making tissues more accessible to the active ingredient, such as collagenase [52].

R-lyase is an enzyme that degrades different glycosaminoglycans, breaking the beta-bonds of 1,4-N-acetylglucosaminidase, which increases the permeability of skin and connective tissues. Lyases have been described and used in techniques such as mesotherapy to correct excesses or complications after the application of injectable gels containing hyaluronic acid, to increase the action of local anesthesia, to prevent the risk of necrosis in sclerotherapy and for their fibrinolytic action [53].

It has been observed that the majority of hard to heal wounds (60%) requiring debridement are associated with biofilms, while only 6% of acute wounds were characterized as containing biofilms [54]. Clinically, biofilms delay healing in several types of chronic wounds [55, 56]. Studies of the interaction between bacteria and wound tissue in keratinocyte cultures *in vitro* and in animal wound models *in vivo* have further validated the causal role of biofilms in chronic wounds [57, 58]. Therefore, the presence of biofilms in chronic wounds is crucial to formulate a clinical treatment plan.

Lyase enzymes act by degrading the ECM of biofilms, altering their structure and making bacteria more susceptible to antimicrobial agents and host defenses. Several studies have investigated the use of lyase enzymes, alone or in combination with other treatments, to alter biofilms in hard to heal wounds [59]. A recent study shows that the purified marine alginate lyase enzyme (AlyP1400) is able to degrade biofilms of *Pseudomonas aeruginosa* biofilms and enhances the bactericidal activity of the antibiotic tobramycin, while modulating the expression of genes related to resistance to efflux antibiotics: bdlA, mexF, mexY, and ndvB, suggesting the increased susceptibility of *P. aeruginosa* biofilms to efflux antibiotics [60].

Hyaluronic acid is a glycosaminoglycan that is one of the components of connective tissues. It is the main constituent of the ECM in the skin, which also plays an important role in the tissue regeneration process [31]. Hyaluronic acid maintains structures to support the biological function of organs and has a strong ability to retain water on the wound surface, which can prevent dryness of injured sites and promote the speed of healing [61].

Hyaluronic acid has anti-inflammatory properties that can help reduce inflammation in the wound, which contributes to faster and more effective healing. Hyaluronic acid acts as a mechanical barrier (anti-adherent gel) that allows debridement in hypertrophic scars, but also inhibits the increase of tumor growth factor beta (TGF-β), an important factor in fibrosis. This allows a decrease in the inflammatory response in wounds (another factor contributing to fibrosis) and the formation of erratic collagen fibers allowing it to organize and distribute in healthy tissue patterns [62, 63].

The presence of hyaluronic acid is very important for tissue hydration and elasticity due to its physicochemical characteristics. The extracellular and homogeneous arrangement of hyaluronic acid throughout the dermal tissue in normal skin, as well as in fine scar fibrosis, appears to play a key role in tissue normalization and in the proper formation of new fibrillar structures.

Hyaluronic acid has been used as a wound treatment due to its unique properties that promote healing. El-Aassar et al. fabricated hyaluronic acid/polygalacturonic acid nano-fibrous mats embedded with silver nanoparticles; an *in vivo* study showed that maximum wound epithelialization and collagen deposition were achieved after 14 days, indicating its effective use for rapid healing of wound infections [64]. Hyaluronan may also play a role in controlling angiogenesis. High-molecular-weight hyaluronan from the extracellular matrix has been shown to inhibit angiogenesis [65, 66].

7.2 Lipase

Lipases (or glycerol ester hydrolases) are a group of enzymes that catalyze the reversible hydrolysis of triglycerides to free fatty acids and glycerol [23]. The role of lipases in the healing process is still under investigation, but their expression has been found to be closely linked to the function of neutrophils, macrophages, and myofibroblasts [67]. Research on defects in adipogenesis has revealed that fat tissue plays an important role during skin repair. The presence of functional adipocytes is necessary for fibroblast recruitment to wounds. Furthermore, although adipogenesis-defective mice produce normal epithelialization, the scar formed is unstable due to fibroblast dysfunction secondary to the lack of necessary adipocyte signaling. Additionally, transplantation of fat tissue-derived mesenchymal cells into wounds causes a shift in macrophage cytokine secretion from pro-inflammatory to anti-inflammatory [68].

This enzymatic treatment associated with hyaluronic acid (PBSERUM SHS30 and PBSERUM HA 2.0 HIGH) plays a key role in breaking down protein barriers that hinder progression to the proliferative phase and promoting a more favorable microenvironment for healing. It is generally assumed, based on available evidence, that all chronic wounds contain biofilm.

The TIMERS consensus has defined a therapeutic pathway for addressing biofilm, which is "based on early intervention under the assumption of its presence, with a series of de-escalation steps aimed at removing as much biofilm as possible and preventing its recurrence." From approximately day one to day four, multimodal therapies should be implemented, including: aggressive debridement when indicated, topical antimicrobials targeting biofilm, and systemic antibiotics. Systemic antibiotics must always be supported by microbiological data obtained in surgical settings.

In 1 week, the response to treatment should be assessed, along with further debridement as needed and the initiation of personalized antimicrobial therapy. As the wound improves, treatment is gradually de-escalated during approximately 4 weeks. During this de-escalation phase, inflammation and healing are evaluated, maintenance debridement is performed, the antimicrobial strategy is reassessed, and the host factors are managed.

The pathway may follow different trajectories from week four onward, depending on the clinical response, until full closure—if that is the established goal of care. When the wound shows potential for closure, the SoC is continued. When the wound shows no signs of closure, as evidenced by lack of size reduction, treatment is intensified.

If a maintenance or palliative approach is to be followed, the entire interdisciplinary team must be involved in any decision to initiate palliative care for the patient.

The growing burden of chronic wounds, postoperative complications has created an urgent need for more efficient, accessible, and continuous monitoring strategies in clinical care. Traditional approaches, often reliant on in-person assessments, are limited by subjectivity, logistical barriers, and delays in detecting complications. In this context, artificial intelligence (AI) has emerged as a transformative tool, enabling a paradigm shift in wound management through real-time analysis, remote surveillance, and predictive decision-making. Recent innovations are leveraging the synergy between AI, mobile applications, and smart sensors to enhance the accuracy and efficiency of wound evaluation while reducing patient burden and healthcare costs. These systems aim not only to digitize clinical observation but to empower both clinicians and patients with actionable insights.

One notable example of this technological shift is RedScar©, an application developed for the remote monitoring of postoperative abdominal wounds. In a study involving 47 patients, it achieved 100% sensitivity and 83% specificity for detecting infections, with near-perfect agreement with clinical evaluations (κ = 0.817). In a similar vein, WoundAIssist, launched in June 2025, integrates on-device AI for wound segmentation, interactive questionnaires, and virtual clinician communication. Designed specifically for elderly users at home, it demonstrated high usability and patient engagement. Additionally, the Multi-Analyte Swab Monitoring system, an experimental tool introduced in May 2025, combines sensor-enabled swabs with an iOS application that analyzes pre- and post-contact images of the wound area, enabling automated assessments of healing progression [69].

Together, these initiatives highlight a clear trend toward multimodal monitoring models that integrate clinical images, biosensors, and remote data acquisition. These approaches are proving effective in the early detection of wound complications and improving therapeutic oversight. However, several challenges remain, including the need for large, diverse datasets, thorough clinical validation, process standardization, and the development of responsible human-AI interfaces. Additionally, ensuring algorithmic transparency and robust data privacy safeguards is essential to secure their ethical and reliable integration into clinical practice [70].

8. Modifying the care pathway and referring if necessary to specialists or MDT

Comprehensive patient assessment, encompassing the local condition of the foot, metabolic, mental, and emotional status, as well as the aforementioned classification systems, forms the foundation for individualized, needs-based therapeutic decision-making. This approach allows for the identification of two main groups: those who can be managed on an outpatient basis, as they do not require continuous or inpatient monitoring, and those who require hospitalization for ongoing observation due to the need for invasive procedures or the management of comorbidities associated with their primary condition.

Traditionally, the Society for Vascular Surgery has used the Fontaine and Rutherford systems to assess the risk of amputation and the potential benefit of revascularization, classifying patients into two key groups: those with ischemic rest pain and those with tissue loss (see **Table 7**). However, the rise in the number of patients with type 2 diabetes mellitus in the recent decades has complicated the direct application of this classification to individuals presenting with an acute diabetic foot condition.

The interdisciplinary management of these patients is essential to optimize outcomes and prevent adverse events that perpetuate pain. The care team must include nursing, general or chronic care medicine, internal medicine, orthopedics, vascular surgery, physical medicine and rehabilitation, infectious diseases, and psychology, among others.

Once the patient has been evaluated and classified according to their current condition, an individualized interdisciplinary management plan is defined.

In this context, patients classified in Fontaine stages I and IIa—those who are asymptomatic or have non-disabling claudication—can generally continue with the outpatient management, provided that regular follow-up appointments are scheduled with the relevant specialties according to their stage. This includes wound or non-infected ulcer care, vascular surgery follow-up, orthopedics, and internal medicine for the management of underlying conditions and complication prevention. It is important to note that even asymptomatic patients may present with concomitant conditions that mask symptoms. Therefore, in older adults or individuals with a history or suspicion of neuropathy, as

Stage	Symptoms
I	Asymptomatic
II A	Non-disabling claudication
II B	Disabling claudication
III	Ischemic rest pain

Table 7.
Fontaine & Rutherford classification.

well as those with reduced mobility due to other conditions, a detailed gait assessment is recommended to confirm their asymptomatic status.

To achieve effective outpatient control in these patients, clear and objective goals (see **Table 1**) have been established, serving as a shared framework for all specialties involved in their care. This strategy emphasizes the importance of coordinated communication and illustrates how a comprehensive approach to the patient significantly contributes to their recovery. When a goal is not done, a timely referral to other specialties becomes a priority action to optimize the patient's comprehensive management. For diabetic patients, the inclusion of endocrinology and nephrology in the care team is critical to address the specific aspects of their disease and thus increase the chances of achieving treatment goals.

In contrast, there is a group of patients for whom hospitalization becomes imminent. This includes those requiring urgent or priority evaluation by specialties such as vascular surgery, orthopedics, intensive care, and internal medicine. These patients typically either fail to meet previously established therapeutic goals or present with progressive clinical deterioration despite outpatient management. Criteria such as abscess, compartment syndrome, necrosis, sepsis, need for drainage or resection, amputation, and ischemia should be considered to identify candidates for interdisciplinary consultation or those who require continuous medical supervision.

Interdisciplinary assessment is essential to accurately classify the current state of the diabetic foot, distinguishing whether the condition is an infectious and ischemic process or if each pathology presents independently. It is crucial to recognize that various manifestations—such as a necrotic foot or an ulcer (i.e., Fontaine stage IV or Saint Elian stage III, respectively)—make ablative procedures a viable option for infection control and management of systemic infections or generalized metabolic decompensation.

The management of hard-to-heal wounds secondary to poorly controlled or difficult-to-manage diabetes mellitus is not performed on an outpatient basis. The diabetic pathophysiology impairs normal wound healing, prolonging healing times already extended compared to non-diabetic individuals and increasing risk for infection. In this context, advanced wound healing techniques are critically important for controlling complications. As a general rule, necrotic tissue should be debrided prior to initiating pro-healing therapies, as the presence of devitalized tissue hinders the effectiveness of such treatments.

9. Patient/family education throughout the SoC

Education should be provided throughout the entire care pathway. In brief, the level of the patient's understanding of their condition and their ability to learn about it and its care

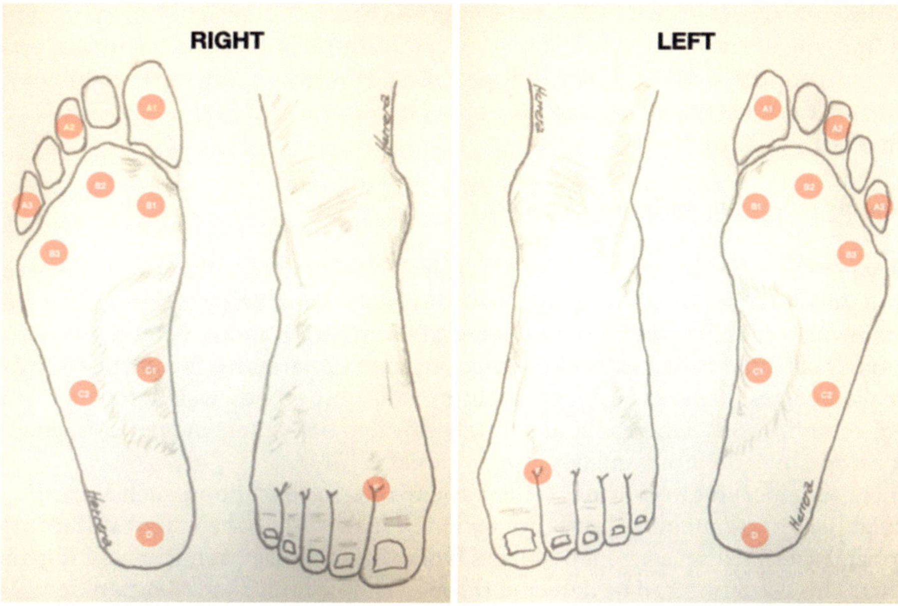

Figure 1.
Diabetic foot examination sites with Semmes Weinstein 5.07 (10-gr.) monofilaments and coding of each site. Reproduced with permission from Herrera-Arbelaez JM, available at: htttps://www.drherreradelpie.com/protopacientes/piediabetico.pdf

should be determined. Specialized centers in diabetic foot care usually have guidelines to patients published on a website or printed available for patients and their relatives or support groups. Most important than anything else, is no to admit these kind of patients in services or offices that are not used to manage these kinds of pathology or even worse, delay a referral trying to achieve a successful outcome on managing a hard to heal wound after 4 weeks when the improvement criteria are not yet fulfilled.

Periodic evaluation offers a crucial opportunity to educate the patient, emphasizing that the wound is not an isolated event, but rather a manifestation of a metabolic disease. Actively involving the patient in their self-care through an educational approach focused on prevention, continuous monitoring, and therapeutic adherence helps improve both functional outcomes and overall quality of life [69].

It is always important to instruct the patient, relatives, or support group to perform a self-examination of sensation with Semmes-Weinstein monofilaments (5.07/10gr) and record all negative spots as (−) in a form following the correct notation (see **Figure 1**).

Progression of neuropathy usually comes from distal to proximal and from medial (medial plantar nerve) to lateral (lateral plantar nerve). A heel absent (−) sensation means posterior tibial compromise above the ankle (Baxter nerve) and a dorsal 1st interdigital space (−) means common sciatic nerve compromise proximal in the calf.

10. Discharge or transition to maintenance treatment to prevent recurrence

Diabetic foot represents one of the most serious complications of diabetes mellitus, characterized by infections, chronic ulcers, and a high risk of amputation.

Multidisciplinary management has proven to be effective in reducing complications and improving clinical outcomes, integrating the efforts of physicians, nurses, podiatrists, nutritionists, and rehabilitation specialists. However, challenges remain in organizing these teams, incorporating new technologies, and adapting care to diverse settings [70].

10.1 Comprehensive patient assessment

Beyond the wound itself, the patient's overall condition significantly influences the progression of lesions. Parameters such as glycated hemoglobin (HbA1c), serum albumin, and renal function provide essential information about metabolic control, infection risk, and healing capacity. Moreover, nutritional status is directly linked to clinical outcomes: patients with hypoalbuminemia or low body weight have a higher risk of complications, whereas a moderately elevated body mass index (BMI) may offer certain metabolic advantages in specific cases [71, 72].

It is also important to consider other patient-related conditions, such as cardiovascular health and mobility levels. Many individuals with diabetic foot suffer from peripheral arterial disease, which reduces blood flow to the extremities and impairs healing. This condition can be detected through simple tools such as the ankle-brachial index (ABI), and in more complex cases, through vascular imaging studies. Additionally, the presence of frailty, sarcopenia, or functional decline—particularly in older adults—may compromise treatment response and increase the risk of new lesions. Therefore, looking beyond the wound and integrating these clinical variables into the initial assessment allows for the design of more realistic, personalized, and effective treatment strategies.

Physical therapy should focus on recovering unconscious proprioception, aiming for a result of 20–40 seconds in the Herrera proprioception test. Achieving this goal typically involves management through physical therapy modalities, including galvanic current stimulation (which is more effective than TENS), areas affected by neuropathy, and manual lymphatic drainage exercises to reduce edema.

Although patient education is generally similar to that provided for hard-to-heal wounds in terms of maintaining overall health, it must be emphasized that a recurrence should never be waited for again.

To prevent recurrence, an annual evaluation by both ophthalmology and orthopedics (foot and ankle surgery) must be performed. Both specialties should remember the mutual and mandatory annual referral of the patient as to "Keep an eye on diabetic foot".

11. Record actions/outcomes at every episode of care

In general, the Saint Elian and TIMERS classification and prognostic tools are used to document each care encounter. Records must be meticulous and should be completed during every consultation, visit, or dressing change.

Author details

Juan Manuel Herrera-Arbelaez*, Diego Morales-Suarez, Carolina Fonseca, Pascual Bernal-Ovalle and Daniel Santiago Cortés-Sarmiento
Muscle-Skeletal Basic and Clinical Research Group, Orthopedic Residency Program-Universidad El Bosque, Bogotá D.C., Colombia

*Address all correspondence to: jmherreraarbelaez@gmail.com

References

[1] Guest JF, Fuller GW, Vowden P. Diabetic foot ulcer management in clinical practice in the UK: Costs and outcomes. International Wound Journal. 2018;**15**(1):43-52. DOI: 10.1111/iwj.12816

[2] Guest JF, Fuller GW, Vowden P. Venous leg ulcer management in clinical practice in the UK: Costs and outcomes. International Wound Journal. 2018;**15**(1):29-37. DOI: 10.1111/iwj.12814

[3] Atkin L, Bućko Z, Conde Montero E, Cutting K, Moffatt C, Probst A, et al. Implementing TIMERS: The race against hard-to-heal wounds. Journal of Wound Care. 2019;**23**(Sup3a):S1-S50. DOI: 10.12968/jowc.2019.28.Sup3a.S1

[4] Wing RR, Lang W, Wadden TA, Safford M, Knowler WC, Bertoni AG, et al. Benefits of modest weight loss in improving cardiovascular risk factors in overweight and obese individuals with type 2 diabetes. Diabetes Care. 2011;**34**(7):1481-1486. DOI: 10.2337/dc10-2415

[5] Gibbons CH, Freeman R. Treatment-induced neuropathy of diabetes: An acute, iatrogenic complication of diabetes. Brain. 2015;**138**(Pt 1):43-52. DOI: 10.1093/brain/awu307

[6] Guo W, Zhou Q, Jia Y, Xu J. Increased levels of glycated hemoglobin A1c and iron deficiency anemia: A review. Medical Science Monitor. 2019;**25**:8371-8378. DOI: 10.12659/MSM.916719

[7] Kazamel M, Stino AM, Smith AG. Metabolic syndrome and peripheral neuropathy. Muscle & Nerve. 2021;**63**(3):285-293. DOI: 10.1002/mus.27086

[8] Lampropoulou IT, Stangou M, Papagianni A, Didangelos T, Iliadis F, Efstratiadis G. TNF-α and microalbuminuria in patients with type 2 diabetes mellitus. Journal Diabetes Research. 2014;**2014**:394206. DOI: 10.1155/2014/394206

[9] Gæde P, Oellgaard J, Carstensen B, Rossing P, Lund-Andersen H, Parving HH, et al. Years of life gained by multifactorial intervention in patients with type 2 diabetes mellitus and microalbuminuria: 21 years follow-up on the Steno-2 randomised trial. Diabetologia. 2016;**59**(11):2298-2307. DOI: 10.1007/s00125-016-4065-6

[10] Galeano-Fernández TF, Carretero-Gómez J, Vidal-Ríos AS, García-García GM, García-Carrasco C, Monreal-Periañez FJ, et al. Impact of diabetes, malnutrition and sarcopenia on the prognosis of patients admitted to internal medicine. Revista Clínica Española (English Edition) (Barcelona). 2023;**223**(9):523-531. DOI: 10.1016/j.rceng.2023.09.004

[11] Ramsey DJ, Kwan JT, Sharma A. Keeping an eye on the diabetic foot: The connection between diabetic eye disease and wound healing in the lower extremity. World Journal of Diabetes. 2022;**13**(12):1035-1048. DOI: 10.4239/wjd.v13.i12.1035

[12] Triana-Ricci R, Martinez-de-Jesus F, Aragón-Carreno MP, et al. Management recommendations for diabetic foot patients. Instructional course. Revista Colombiana de Ortopedia y Traumatología. 2021;**35**(4):330-357. DOI: 10.1016/j.rccot.2022.02.001

[13] Armstrong DG, Boulton AJM, Bus SA. Diabetic foot ulcers and their recurrence. The New England Journal of Medicine. 2017;**376**:2367-2375. DOI: 10.1056/NEJMra1615439

[14] Gallagher KA, Mills JL, Armstrong DG, Conte MS, Kirsner RS, Minc SD, et al. Current status and principles for the treatment and prevention of diabetic foot ulcers in the cardiovascular patient population: A scientific statement from the American Heart Association. Circulation. 2024;**149**(4):e232-e253. DOI: 10.1161/CIR.0000000000001192

[15] Fitridge R, Thompson MM, editors. Mechanisms of Vascular Disease: A Textbook for Vascular Surgeons. Adelaide: University of Adelaide Press; 2023

[16] Rincón Y, Gil V, Pacheco J, Benítez I, Sánchez M. Evaluación y tratamiento del pie diabético. Revista venezolana de endocrinología y metabolismo. 2012;**10**(3):8-15

[17] Escobar C, Sánchez-Bautista P, Romero-Ramos M, et al. Clasificación de San Elian: una herramienta para el pronóstico funcional del pie diabético. Revista Colombiana de Cirugía. 2021;**36**(4):289-296

[18] Falanga V. Wound healing and its impairment in the diabetic foot. Lancet. 2005;**366**(9498):1736-1743. DOI: 10.1016/S0140-6736(05)67700-8

[19] Guo S, Dipietro LA. Factors affecting wound healing. Journal of Dental Research. 2010;**89**(3):219-229. DOI: 10.1177/0022034509359125

[20] Bainbridge P. Wound healing and the role of fibroblasts. Journal of Wound Care. 2013;**22**(8):407-408, 410-412. DOI: 10.12968/jowc.2013.22.8.407

[21] Jude EB, Eleftheriadou I, Tentolouris N. Peripheral arterial disease in diabetes--a review. Diabetic Medicine. 2010;**27**(1):4-14. DOI: 10.1111/j.1464-5491.2009.02866.x

[22] Hingorani A, LaMuraglia GM, Henke P, Meissner MH, Loretz L, Zinszer KM, et al. The management of diabetic foot: A clinical practice guideline by the Society for Vascular Surgery in collaboration with the American Podiatric Medical Association and the Society for Vascular Medicine. Journal of Vascular Surgery. 2016;**63**(2 Suppl):3S-21S. DOI: 10.1016/j.jvs.2015.10.003

[23] Vinik AI. Diabetic neuropathy: Pathogenesis and therapy. The American Journal of Medicine. 1999;**107**(2B):17S-26S. DOI: 10.1016/s0002-9343(99)00009-1

[24] Boulton AJ. The pathway to foot ulceration in diabetes. The Medical Clinics of North America. 2013;**97**(5):775-790. DOI: 10.1016/j.mcna.2013.03.007

[25] Faglia E. Characteristics of peripheral arterial disease and its relevance to the diabetic population. The International Journal of Lower Extremity Wounds. 2011;**10**(3):152-166. DOI: 10.1177/1534734611417352

[26] Shy ME, Frohman EM, So YT, Arezzo JC, Cornblath DR, Giuliani MJ, et al. Quantitative sensory testing: Report of the Therapeutics and Technology Assessment Subcommittee of the American Academy of Neurology. Neurology. 2003;**60**(6):898-904. DOI: 10.1212/01.wnl.0000058546.16985.11

[27] Hu A, Koh B, Teo MR. A review of the current evidence on the sensitivity and specificity of the Ipswich touch test for the screening of loss of protective sensation in patients with diabetes mellitus. Diabetology International. 2020;**12**(2):145-150. DOI: 10.1007/s13340-020-00451-9

[28] Hernández N, Álvarez G, Bravo F, Vieira JC, Reina EA, Herrera JM.

Validación de la prueba de Romberg Modificada para la determinación del tiempo de propiocepción inconciente en adultos sanos. Revista Colombiana de Ortopedia y Traumatología. 2018;**32**(2):93-99. DOI: 10.1016/j.rccot.2017.11.001

[29] Mascio A, Comisi C, Cinelli V, Pitocco D, Greco T, Maccauro G, et al. Radiological assessment of Charcot neuro-osteoarthropathy in diabetic foot: A narrative review. Diagnostics (Basel). 2025;**15**(6):767. DOI: 10.3390/diagnostics15060767

[30] Arias-Alvarez M, Gella L, Arimany-Manso J, Cardoner M, Hernández C, Simó R, et al. Electrophysiological findings in long-term type 1 diabetes patients without diabetic retinopathy using different ERG recording systems. Scientific Reports. 2024;**14**:3520. DOI: 10.1038/s41598-024-54099-5

[31] Balla T, Nagy Z, Kiss HJ, Gombos K. Further evidence for the utility of electrophysiological methods for the detection of subclinical retinal and optic nerve involvement in diabetes. Ophthalmic Research. 2017;**57**(3):196-204. DOI: 10.1159/000455324

[32] Kumar A, Jahan F, Rizvi SMA. Visual evoked potentials for the detection of diabetic retinal neuropathy. International Journal of Molecular Sciences. 2023;**24**(8):7361. DOI: 10.3390/ijms24087361

[33] Barnes JA, Eid MA, Creager MA, Goodney PP. Epidemiology and risk of amputation in patients with diabetes mellitus and peripheral artery disease. Arteriosclerosis, Thrombosis, and Vascular Biology. 2020;**40**(8):1808-1817. DOI: 10.1161/ATVBAHA.120.314595

[34] Hinchliffe RJ, Brownrigg JR, Apelqvist J, Boyko EJ, Fitridge R, Mills JL, et al. IWGDF guidance on the diagnosis, prognosis and management of peripheral artery disease in patients with foot ulcers in diabetes. Diabetes/Metabolism Research and Reviews. 2016;**32**(Suppl. 1):37-44. DOI: 10.1002/dmrr.2698

[35] Soyoye DO, Abiodun OO, Ikem RT, Kolawole BA, Akintomide AO. Diabetes and peripheral artery disease: A review. World Journal of Diabetes. 2021;**12**(6):827-838. DOI: 10.4239/wjd.v12.i6.827

[36] Khanna S, Biswas S, Shang Y, et al. Macrophage dysfunction impairs resolution of inflammation in the wounds of diabetic mice. PLoS One. 2010;**5**(3):e9539. DOI: 10.1371/journal.pone.0009539

[37] Clayton SM, Shafikhani SH, Soulika AM. Macrophage and neutrophil dysfunction in diabetic wounds. Advances in Wound Care (New Rochelle). 2024;**13**(9):463-484. DOI: 10.1089/wound.2023.0149

[38] Callaghan MJ, Ceradini DJ, Gurtner GC. Hyperglycemia-induced reactive oxygen species and impaired endothelial progenitor cell function. Antioxidants & Redox Signaling. 2005;**7**(11-12):1476-1482. DOI: 10.1089/ars.2005.7.1476

[39] Stechmiller JK. Understanding the role of nutrition and wound healing. Nutrition in Clinical Practice. 2010;**25**(1):61-68. DOI: 10.1177/0884533609358997

[40] Gonzalez JS, Tanenbaum ML, Commissariat PV. Psychosocial factors in medication adherence and diabetes self-management: Implications for research and practice. The American Psychologist. 2016;**71**(7):539-551. DOI: 10.1037/a0040388

[41] Feil DG, Zhu CW, Sultzer DL. The relationship between cognitive impairment and diabetes self-management in a population-based community sample of older adults with type 2 diabetes. Journal of Behavioral Medicine. 2012;**35**(2):190-199. DOI: 10.1007/s10865-011-9344-6

[42] Ding JY, Chen MJ, Wu LF, Shu GF, Fang SJ, Li ZY, et al. Mesenchymal stem cell-derived extracellular vesicles in skin wound healing: Roles, opportunities and challenges. Military Medical Research. 2023;**10**:36. DOI: 10.1186/s40779-023-00472-w

[43] Yang J, Chen Z, Pan D, Li H, Shen J. Umbilical cord-derived mesenchymal stem cell-derived exosomes combined pluronic F127 hydrogel promote chronic diabetic wound healing and complete skin regeneration. International Journal of Nanomedicine. 2020;**15**:5911-5926. DOI: 10.2147/IJN.S249129

[44] Shah SA, Sohail M, Khan S, Minhas MU, de Matas M, Sikstone V, et al. Biopolymer-based biomaterials for accelerated diabetic wound healing: A critical review. International Journal of Biological Macromolecules. 2019;**139**:975-993. DOI: 10.1016/j.ijbiomac.2019.08.007

[45] Aldahish A, Shanmugasundaram N, Vasudevan R, Alqahtani T, Alqahtani S, Mohammad Asiri A, et al. Silk fibroin nanofibers: Advancements in bioactive dressings through electrospinning technology for diabetic wound healing. Pharmaceuticals (Basel). 2024;**17**(10):1305. DOI: 10.3390/ph17101305

[46] Tian Z, Chen H, Zhao P. Compliant immune response of silk-based biomaterials broadens application in wound treatment. Frontiers in Pharmacology. 2025;**16**:1548837. DOI: 10.3389/fphar.2025.1548837

[47] Camargo J, Vanegas N, Velez JD, Lopez JC, Herrera-Arbelaez JM. Plasma rico en plaquetas (PRP) como sistema de entrega local de antibióticos en infecciones óseas: estudio in vitro. Revista Colombiana de Ortopedia y Traumatología. 2012;**26**(1):39-49

[48] Escobar J, Castro B, Vanegas N, Leon LJ, Velez JD, Camargo J, et al. Evaluación cualitativa y cuantitativa *in vitro* del gel de plasma rico en plaquetas (PRP) como sistema de entrega local de antibióticos. Revista Colombiana de Ortopedia y Traumatología. 2015;**29**(4):146-151. DOI: 10.1016/j.rccot.2016.03.003

[49] Daboor SM, Budge SM, Ghaly AE, Brooks SL, Dave D. Extraction and purification of collagenase enzymes: A critical review. American Journal of Biochemistry and Biotechnology. 2010;**6**:239-263. DOI: 10.3844/ajbbsp.2010.239.263

[50] Jeffcoate WJ, Price P, Harding KG, International Working Group on Wound Healing and Treatments for People with Diabetic Foot Ulcers. Wound healing and treatments for people with diabetic foot ulcers. Diabetes/Metabolism Research and Reviews. 2004;**20**(Suppl. 1):S78-S89. DOI: 10.1002/dmrr.476

[51] Bitencourt CS, Pereira PA, Ramos SG, Sampaio SV, Arantes EC, Aronoff DM, et al. Hyaluronidase recruits mesenchymal-like cells to the lung and ameliorates fibrosis. Fibrogenesis & Tissue Repair. 2011;**4**(1):3. DOI: 10.1186/1755-1536-4-3

[52] Fierro-Arias L et al. Enzymatic products (hyaluronidase, collagenase and lipase) in dermatology. Dermatologia Revista Mexicana. *2017*;**63**:206-219

[53] James GA, Swogger E, Wolcott R, Ed P, Secor P, Sestrich J, et al. Biofilms

in chronic wounds. Wound Repair and Regeneration. 2008;**16**(1):37-44. DOI: 10.1111/j.1524-475X.2007.00321.x

[54] Metcalf DG, Bowler PG. Biofilm delays wound healing: A review of the evidence. Burns Trauma. 2013;**1**(1):5-12. DOI: 10.4103/2321-3868.113329

[55] Hurlow J, Bowler PG. Potential implications of biofilm in chronic wounds: A case series. Journal of Wound Care. 2012;**21**(3):109-110. 112, 114 passim. DOI: 10.12968/jowc.2012.21.3.109

[56] Price LB, Liu CM, Melendez JH, Frankel YM, Engelthaler D, Aziz M, et al. Community analysis of chronic wound bacteria using 16S rRNA gene-based pyrosequencing: Impact of diabetes and antibiotics on chronic wound microbiota. PLoS One. 2009;**4**(7):e6462. DOI: 10.1371/journal.pone.0006462

[57] Zhao G, Usui ML, Underwood RA, Singh PK, James GA, Stewart PS, et al. Time course study of delayed wound healing in a biofilm-challenged diabetic mouse model. Wound Repair and Regeneration. 2012;**20**(3):342-352. DOI: 10.1111/j.1524-475X.2012.00793.x

[58] Wang S, Zhao Y, Breslawec AP, Liang T, Deng Z, Kuperman LL, et al. Strategy to combat biofilms: A focus on biofilm dispersal enzymes. npj Biofilms and Microbiomes. 2023;**9**(1):63. DOI: 10.1038/s41522-023-00427-y

[59] Daboor SM, Raudonis R, Cheng Z. Characterizations of the viability and gene expression of dispersal cells from *Pseudomonas aeruginosa* biofilms released by alginate lyase and tobramycin. PLoS One. 2021;**16**(10):e0258950. DOI: 10.1371/journal.pone.0258950

[60] Catanzano O, D'Esposito V, Acierno S, Ambrosio MR, De Caro C, Avagliano C, et al. Alginate-hyaluronan composite hydrogels accelerate wound healing process. Carbohydrate Polymers. 2015;**131**:407-414. DOI: 10.1016/j.carbpol.2015.05.081

[61] Aduba DC, Yang H. Polysaccharide fabrication platforms and biocompatibility assessment as candidate wound dressing materials. Bioengineering (Basel). 2017;**4**(1):1. DOI: 10.3390/bioengineering4010001

[62] Ruppert SM, Hawn TR, Arrigoni A, Wight TN, Bollyky PL. Tissue integrity signals communicated by high-molecular weight hyaluronan and the resolution of inflammation. Immunologic Research. 2014;**58**(2-3):186-192. DOI: 10.1007/s12026-014-8495-2

[63] Petrey AC, de la Motte CA. Hyaluronan, a crucial regulator of inflammation. Frontiers in Immunology. 2014;**5**:101. DOI: 10.3389/fimmu.2014.00101

[64] El-Aassar MR, Ibrahim OM, Fouda MMG, El-Beheri NG, Agwa MM. Wound healing of nanofiber comprising polygalacturonic/hyaluronic acid embedded silver nanoparticles: In-vitro and in-vivo studies. Carbohydrate Polymers. 2020;**238**:116175. DOI: 10.1016/j.carbpol.2020.116175

[65] Dvorak HF, Harvey VS, Estrella P, Brown LF, McDonagh J, Dvorak AM. Fibrin containing gels induce angiogenesis. Implications for tumor stroma generation and wound healing. Laboratory Investigation. 1987;**57**(6):673-686

[66] West DC, Kumar S. The effect of hyaluronate and its oligosaccharides on endothelial cell proliferation and monolayer integrity. Experimental Cell Research. 1989;**183**(1):179-196. DOI: 10.1016/0014-4827(89)90428-x

[67] Ma WX, Yu TS, Fan YY, Zhang ST, Ren P, Wang SB, et al. Time-dependent expression and distribution of monoacylglycerol lipase during the skin-incised wound healing in mice. International Journal of Legal Medicine. 2011;**125**(4):549-558. DOI: 10.1007/s00414-011-0567-4

[68] Rivera-Gonzalez G, Shook B, Horsley V. Adipocytes in skin health and disease. Cold Spring Harbor Perspectives in Medicine. 2014;**4**(3):a015271. DOI: 10.1101/cshperspect.a015271

[69] Walburn J, Vedhara K, Hankins M, Rixon L, Weinman J. Psychological stress and wound healing in humans: A systematic review and meta-analysis. Journal of Psychosomatic Research. 2009;**67**(3):253-271. DOI: 10.1016/j.jpsychores.2009.04.002

[70] Craus-Miguel A, Munar M, Moyà-Alcover G, Contreras-Nogales AM, González-Hidalgo M, Segura-Sampedro JJ. Enhancing surgical wound monitoring: A paired cohort study evaluating a new AI-based application for automatic detection of potential infections. Journal of Clinical Medicine. 2024;**13**(24):7863. DOI: 10.3390/jcm13247863

[71] Kaiser MJ, Bauer JM, Ramsch C, Uter W, Guigoz Y, Cederholm T, et al. Validation of the mini nutritional assessment short-form (MNA-SF): A practical tool for identification of nutritional status. The Journal of Nutrition, Health & Aging. 2009;**13**(9):782-788. DOI: 10.1007/s12603-009-0214-7

[72] Dent E, Morley JE, Cruz-Jentoft AJ, Arai H, Kritchevsky SB, Guralnik J, et al. International clinical practice guidelines for sarcopenia (ICFSR): Screening, diagnosis and management. The Journal of Nutrition, Health & Aging. 2018;**22**(10):1148-1161. DOI: 10.1007/s12603-018-1139-9

Section 3

Enzymatic and Biophysical Therapies

Chapter 4

Enzymatic Debridement in Burns: Methods, Indications, Contraindications, and Results

Mihaela Pertea

Abstract

Enzymatic debridement for the treatment of moderate- and deep-thickness burns has seen rapid global uptake in recent years. This growing interest stems from the high selectivity of proteolytic enzymes in removing only non-viable tissue, in contrast to conventional surgical methods. Bromelain—extracted from both the fruit and stem of *Ananas comosus*—has proven exceptionally effective in enzymatic debridement. It is a composite of proteolytic enzymes and non-enzymatic constituents exhibiting anti-inflammatory, fibrinolytic, anti-oedematous, antithrombotic, analgesic, and immunomodulatory properties. The advantages of bromelain-based enzymatic debridement, marketed as NexoBrid® (NXB; MediWound Ltd., Yavne, Israel), have led to its incorporation into treatment protocols for deep burns, challenging the historical gold standard of surgical excision followed by precise grafting. National and European consensus guidelines—as well as numerous reports worldwide—have demonstrated the efficacy of enzymatic debridement (ED) in both adults and children. This study have precisely defined the indications, application technique, contraindications, and anatomical-region-specific considerations for enzymatic debridement, tailored to burn aetiology and depth.

Keywords: burns, enzymatic debridement, bromelain, epitelisation, skin grafts

1. Introduction

Burns cause irreversible protein denaturation in the skin. Thermal injury acts on the skin, most conspicuously on collagen, with consequent disruption of its native triple-helical architecture. This conformational collapse is observed within a narrow thermal window—60 to 65°C—after which the denatured collagen matrix becomes highly susceptible to subsequent proteolytic degradation [1].

Tangential excision of the burn eschar within the first 48 hours after injury represents a critical intervention in the management of partial- and full-thickness burns. Early removal of devitalised tissue significantly diminishes the risks of microbial colonisation, invasive infection, and sepsis, while concurrently shortening the interval to re-epithelialisation and, by extension, the overall length of hospitalisation [2]. The combined approach of tangential excision followed by immediate autologous split-skin grafting was first described by Zora Janzekovic in 1970 and has since become the prevailing therapeutic paradigm for deep dermal and full-thickness burns [3].

Excision of the burn wound can be performed with an electric dermatome, electrocautery, or a conventional scalpel. It is estimated that 30–50% of the excised specimen by these methods often comprises viable, healthy tissue, principally dermis, which is the primary source of epithelial cells essential for spontaneous wound closure [3]. Recognition of the need to conserve this viable dermal matrix has spurred the development of more selective, tissue-sparing modalities. Among surgical selective options, high-speed dermabrasion and hydro-surgical debridement achieve incremental preservation of the dermis, albeit at the cost of prolonged operative times and the requisite use of general anaesthesia [4, 5]. In cases where surgical debridement leaves little or no dermis, immediate coverage of the remaining defect is imperative. The overarching objective to maximise viable tissue preservation has, in turn, catalysed the adoption of non-surgical, selective debridement techniques, which achieve tissue removal without the trauma and sequelae inherent to traditional surgery [6, 7].

2. Debridement

Debridement is the purposeful removal of non-viable tissue, foreign material, contaminated debris, and any bone fragments that may lie within the wound bed. By clearing these barriers, the clinician restores a clean surface and gives the wound the biological conditions it needs to heal. Whatever the underlying cause—thermal, mechanical, vascular, or otherwise—timely debridement remains a cornerstone of modern wound care and an essential prerequisite for reliable closure [8, 9].

Therapeutic wound care unfolds in four inter-locking phases: D – debridement of devitalised tissue; I – control of inflammation and infection; M – optimisation of moisture balance; and E – continual reassessment of the wound micro-environment and progress of epithelialisation. Together, these elements make up the well-established DIME framework, a set of principles embedded in every modern wound-care protocol [10].

The principal aim of debridement is to purge the wound bed of devitalised tissue, thereby creating the physiological conditions required for repair [11]. In addition, debridement is pivotal in disrupting microbial biofilm, removing accumulated biological detritus, and clearing senescent cells that hinder regeneration. Best-practice guidelines therefore advocate performing debridement as early as possible after the inciting trauma—and repeating it serially whenever the wound's appearance or biology warrants—to optimise healing, especially in burn wounds [12, 13].

Debridement is a pivotal step in contemporary wound management because it conditions the wound bed for re-epithelialisation. Devitalised and necrotic tissues provide a nutrient-rich niche for microbial proliferation, thereby amplifying the risk of infection [14]. At the same time, necrotic tissue forms a physical barrier that blocks epithelial migration and prevents topical therapies from reaching viable tissue where they can exert their intended effects [15]. Its continued presence disrupts essential repair mechanisms—including angiogenesis, granulation-tissue formation, epidermal resurfacing, and orderly extracellular-matrix (ECM) remodelling—and can even obscure the clinician's ability to assess the true depth and severity of the lesion, masking incipient or established infection [16]. Taken together, these factors highlight why the prompt and, when necessary, iterative removal of non-viable tissue remains indispensable to optimal wound healing [17]. Over the years, a spectrum of debridement strategies has been described for clearing devitalised tissue: autolytic debridement, biological (larval) debridement, surgical debridement, and enzymatic debridement [18].

2.1 Autolytic debridement

Autolytic debridement is a natural, physiological process in which the body's own phagocytic cells and proteolytic enzymes break down necrotic tissue. Highly selective, it targets only devitalised material and leaves healthy tissue unharmed [19].

Achieving effective autolysis requires a consistently moist wound environment and adequate systemic immune support; moist dressings speed cleansing by softening and loosening areas of necrosis, while irrigation, chemical cleansing, and gentle mechanical debridement further promote detachment of devitalised tissue [20].

The method's efficiency depends on both the amount of necrotic burden and overall wound size, and—being inherently slow—it may take several days to produce visible results. If no meaningful reduction of necrotic tissue is evident after 24–48 hours, an alternative debridement strategy should be considered [20].

2.2 Biological debridement

Biological debridement—more widely recognised as larval therapy—relies on the controlled application of sterile *Lucilia sericata* (green-bottle fly) larvae. The method is particularly advantageous for extensive wounds in which painless removal of necrotic tissue is required [16].

Once placed on the wound bed, the larvae secrete a cocktail of proteolytic enzymes that liquefy non-viable tissue; simultaneously, they ingest the resulting detritus together with resident bacteria, release ammonia that elevates local pH and suppresses microbial growth, and disrupt established biofilms while preventing the formation of new ones—all of which hasten wound resolution [21]. Larvae may be applied directly onto the wound surface or enclosed in a permeable "biobag"; experimental data show that free-range larvae complete debridement in approximately 14 days, twice as fast as biobag-contained larvae ($\approx$ 28 days) and far quicker than autolytic hydrogel dressings ($\approx$72 days) [22].

Contraindications include wounds communicating with the intraperitoneal cavity, lesions of pyoderma gangrenosum in immunosuppressed patients, and ulcers adjacent to joints affected by septic arthritis [21–23].

2.3 Surgical debridement

Surgical debridement encompasses all operative manoeuvres undertaken by the surgeon to excise necrotic tissue from a wound, using instruments such as scalpels, scissors, curettes, and, in the case of burns, electrodermatomes or Watson dermatomes [16, 24].

Because these procedures are inherently painful and often highly haemorrhagic, they must be performed in the operating theatre under strict aseptic conditions and with adequate anaesthesia, which may need to be continued into the immediate postoperative period for optimal patient comfort [25].

Anaesthetic techniques range from general anaesthesia with orotracheal intubation to regional blocks—such as infraclavicular, supraclavicular, or axillary plexus—and spinal anaesthesia, selected according to the location of the wound or burn [16].

Effective postoperative pain control is equally critical and typically combines systemic analgesics and anti-inflammatory agents with prolonged regional anaesthesia when warranted—for example, an epidural catheter when burns involve the lower abdomen, buttocks, or lower limbs, or a continuous peripheral plexus catheter (e.g., Contiplex®) for upper-extremity burns [25]. Surgical debridement inevitably causes bleeding of variable magnitude, so meticulous haemostasis is essential to avert major blood loss and haemodynamic destabilisation. All of these procedures must be carried out by personnel specifically trained in burn surgery and critical care [26].

2.4 Enzymatic debridement

Enzymatic debridement—acknowledged since the 1998 International Society for Burns Injuries (ISBI) meeting in Jerusalem as a "Minimally Invasive Modality" (MIM) of burn care—is distinguished by its high degree of selectivity [27]. The technique employs a proteolytic enzyme to dissolve devitalised tissue while sparing viable structures [28]. Over the years, a variety of protease sources were explored. Ultimately, a bromelain-based preparation that met FDA requirements was developed and approved, and it is now being incorporated increasingly into standard burn care protocols [29].

Current burn care protocols recommend enzymatic debridement for deep partial- and full-thickness injuries of moderate to large extent [30]. Nevertheless, it is contra-indicated in patients with known hypersensitivity to any component of the formulation and in wounds that are already in an advanced reparative stage [31]. It is relatively contra-indicated in heavily infected wounds. In addition, collagenase preparations must not be combined with silver-based dressings or with Dakin's solution, as these agents inactivate the enzyme and nullify its therapeutic effect [32].

3. Enzymatic debridement

3.1 Brief history

Over the decades, many forms of enzymatic debridement have been explored. To identify an agent that is both effective and practical, several benchmark criteria were set: it had to act rapidly and efficiently; be highly selective, leaving intact skin unharmed; contain no allergenic, toxic, or irritant components; possess a chemically stable, easy-to-prepare formulation; and, ideally, be affordable.

Investigators therefore tested a wide array of proteolytic sources.

In the 1950s, Tillett experimented with streptococcal enzymes [33, 34], while Connell introduced a protease called debricin along with other fungal- and bacterial-derived enzymes [35].

In 1951, Altemeier, Hummel, and McMillan evaluated clostridial enzymes from *Clostridium histolyticum* and *Bordetella pertussis* and described a mixed papaya-fruit protease preparation [36]. None of these early efforts produced a clinically viable product, but they paved the way for bromelain-based agents.

In 1957, Heinicke and Gortner isolated a novel protease from pineapple—bromelain—opening a new line of investigation [37].

The following year, Burke and Golden proposed a papaya-enzyme formula combined with urea and chlorophyll, and in the 1960s researchers evaluated proteases obtained from filtrates of *Bacillus subtilis* [38].

Bromelain's therapeutic promise was first demonstrated by Levine in 1971 [39] and later confirmed by Levenson in a porcine burn model [40]; Klein and co-workers likewise reported its efficacy as a burn debriding agent [41, 42].

Building on this body of work, the bromelain-based preparation NexoBrid® received regulatory approval in 2012 as a minimally invasive option for enzymatic debridement of deep partial- and full-thickness burns [43].

The first multicentre study detailing its clinical use in burn care was published by Rosenberg and colleagues, marking its transition into routine practice [44].

3.2 Proteolitic enzymes enriched with bromelain: Nexobrid® (NXB; MediWound Ltd., Yavne, Israel)

Bromelain is an extract derived from the pineapple (*Ananas comosus*), present in both the fruit and the stem. It is a composite of proteolytic enzymes and non-enzymatic constituents whose anti-oedematous, anti-inflammatory, antithrombotic, analgesic, and keratolytic properties have been scientifically validated [45–47].

The mechanisms underlying its activity involve the kallikrein–kinin pathway, arachidonic-acid metabolism, and cell-mediated immune responses [48]. Both fruit bromelain (BAA21848) and stem bromelain (CAA08861) are classified as cysteine proteases; they are active across a pH range of 5.5–8.0 and consist of protease subunits with molecular masses of 20–35 kDa [49].

The anti-inflammatory action of bromelain stems from its modulation of prostaglandins and cytokines, which leads to diminished oedema. In burns, it lowers pro-inflammatory mediators such as TNF-α and select interleukins, thereby reducing swelling, erythema, and pain [48]. By promoting fibrin degradation, it exerts a fibrinolytic effect that enhances local circulation and thus accelerates healing. At the microvascular level, bromelain decreases platelet aggregation, reducing thrombus formation and sustaining tissue perfusion [49]. Antimicrobial activity against *Escherichia coli* and *Staphylococcus aureus* has also been demonstrated, suggesting an additional antibacterial effect [49–51]. Beyond wound care, bromelain is recognised for its mucolytic action in sinusitis and bronchitis and for its role in protein digestion as a component of digestive-enzyme supplements [51].

Although bromelain-based preparations are effective for non-surgical debridement, adequate analgesia is essential during their application, and the surrounding intact skin must be carefully protected [52].

Bromelain selectively digests denatured collagen and necrotic protein matrices without harming nerves, blood vessels, or hair follicles. The bromelain formulation approved in 2012—NexoBrid® (NXB; MediWound Ltd., Yavne, Israel)—contains 0.09 g of bromelain per gram of product. It has secured FDA approval for burn management and is now used widely across Europe and elsewhere [43].

3.3 Indications and method of use of the bromelain-enriched proteolytic enzyme mixture NexoBrid® (NXB; MediWound Ltd., Yavne, Israel)

Peri-operative bromelain therapy has demonstrated efficacy across multiple medical disciplines—including orthopaedics, obstetrics, otorhinolaryngology, dentistry, ophthalmology, sports medicine—and, topically, for the debridement of wounds and burns [43].

Consequently, bromelain constitutes a validated enzymatic alternative to surgical debridement [9, 10]. Enzymatic debridement with NexoBrid® (NXB), a bromelain-enriched proteolytic enzyme mixture, is indicated for patients with deep-partial-thickness (grade II B) and full-thickness (grade III) burns. The original label limited use to adults (>18 years) and to grade II B injuries, but since 2025 NXB has been approved for children of any age, and its indication for grade III burns was endorsed following the 2020 update of the 2017 European consensus [30, 53].

There is no specific age limit that contraindicates the use of enzymatic debridement. This method can be safely employed in the treatment of deep partial-thickness and full-thickness burns caused by scalds, steam, or flames, provided the injury does not extend through the full depth of the skin to the underlying muscle or beyond.

In high-voltage electrical burns, where there is a defined entry and exit point typically represented by deep necrotic lesions, enzymatic debridement may be used in an initial step. However, due to the depth and complexity of these burns—as is also the case with flame burn—enzymatic debridement may need to be followed by surgical debridement and definitive coverage using split-thickness skin grafting.

In chemical burns, whether caused by acids or alkalis, enzymatic debridement is generally not recommended. Despite immediate irrigation with copious amounts of water, chemical agents can remain active for extended periods.

The product used for the enzymatic debridement is supplied in two vials: one containing lyophilised powder and the other a gel vehicle. Reconstitution is achieved by gradually adding the powder to the gel and stirring with a spatula for several minutes until a smooth, lump-free suspension forms; the preparation must be applied to the burn surface within 15 minutes of mixing (**Figure 1**).

Each standard kit provides 2 g of bromelain-enriched concentrate (0.09 g active enzyme per gram of product after reconstitution) suspended in 22 g of gel. A mixture of 2 g powder with 20 g gel treats approximately 1% of total body surface area—about 180 cm^2—while larger vials (5 g powder plus 50 g gel) suffice for roughly 450 cm^2. These calculations assume an application layer 1.5–3 mm thick [7, 43, 54].

The first European consensus on bromelain use in deep-partial and full-thickness burns was adopted in 2017, and NXB has since been incorporated into the standard of care for selected burn types [30]. The consensus recommends application from the first hour up to 72 hours post-injury [30].

Moti Harats et al. later reported favourable outcomes when bromelain was applied between 72 hours and 5 days after the burn [55]. Bromelain has also proved effective in chemical and electrical burns, including paediatric cases; however, its efficacy appears to wane beyond the fifth post-injury day, probably because eschar permeability progressively declines [56].

Initial prescribing guidance limited bromelain application to no more than 15% of total body surface area (TBSA) in a single session, with the option to repeat treatment after 24–48 hours—provided the product is not reapplied to the same anatomical site. The 2017 European consensus on bromelain-based enzymatic debridement (NexoBrid®) was revisited in 2020; the updated statement permits use on any region of the body, including the face, perineum, and genitalia [30, 53].

The most recent (2025) paediatric update allows NexoBrid® at all ages, but restricts treated surface area to ≤15% TBSA in children aged 4–18 years and to ≤10% TBSA in infants and toddlers aged 0–3 years [57].

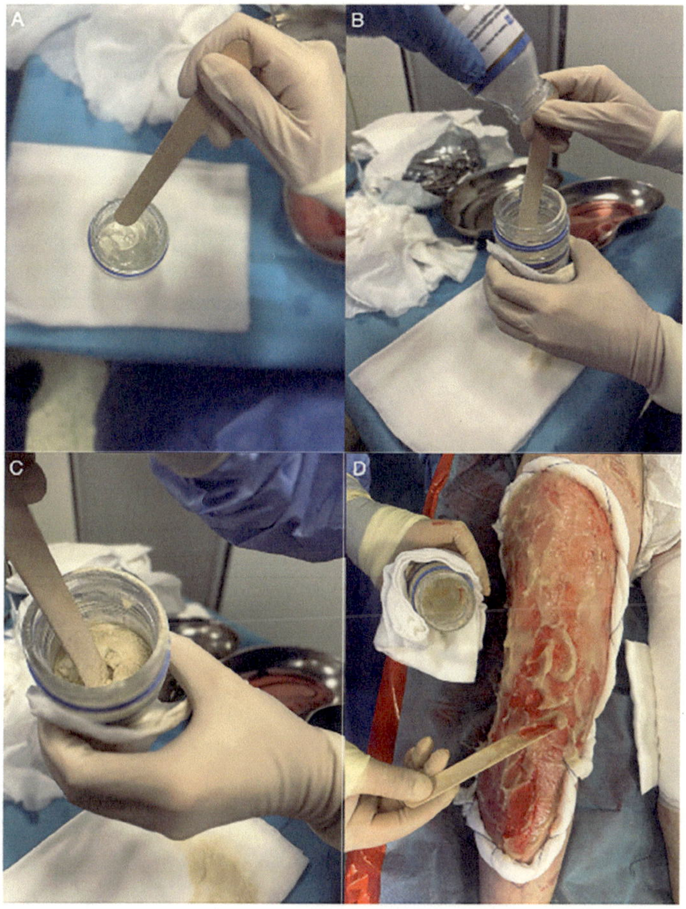

Figure 1.
A. Gel-based vehicle (excipient), B. Combine the gel base with the bromelain powder, C. Thoroughly homogenise the two components (gel/powder), D. Apply the resulting preparation evenly across the burn wound.

3.3.1 Method of application

Although the introduction of NexoBrid® was initially met with scepticism, its clinical value has since been demonstrated in many countries, where it now yields consistently favourable outcomes.

Topical application of the bromelain preparation can reduce—or even eliminate—the need for split-thickness skin grafting by conserving as much viable dermis as possible. The procedure is performed at the patient's bedside, is quick and efficient, and results in substantially less blood loss than conventional surgical debridement [43, 46].

The technical sequence for applying and subsequently removing the debriding agent has been standardised and recommendations for use are made by the manufacturer [58]:

1. *Assessment of burn area and depth*. After obtaining microbiological screening swabs, the burns are irrigated and cleansed with saline. Depth is then determined by clinical examination and, when necessary, echo-Doppler imaging.

Clinical burn assessment and depth grading rely on three bedside cues: skin colour, the presence of blisters, and the nature of their fluid. Clear, straw-coloured serum points to a superficial-partial injury (grade II-A), whereas a sero-sanguinous exudate suggests a deeper partial-thickness burn (II-B degree). Areas of stiff, leathery eschar—brown-black or pearly white—denote a full-thickness injury (grade III).

From a clinical standpoint, depth is refined beyond visual cues by testing capillary refill and revascularisation time and by mapping sensation: a sharp, stinging pain is typical of superficial burns, while dull or absent sensation points to deeper injury. On hair-bearing skin, the "hair-pull test" is informative: in full-thickness burns the follicular bulb is destroyed, so hairs detach with a light wipe of gauze or minimal traction with forceps.

Once burn depth and total surface area have been established, the team decides whether enzymatic debridement is appropriate, taking into account associated injuries, comorbidities, and the patient's current haematological profile.

Echo-Doppler imaging can then corroborate bedside findings, delineating well-perfused zones versus regions of diminished or absent flow, in keeping with the graduated loss of vascularity seen as burns deepen (**Figure 2**).

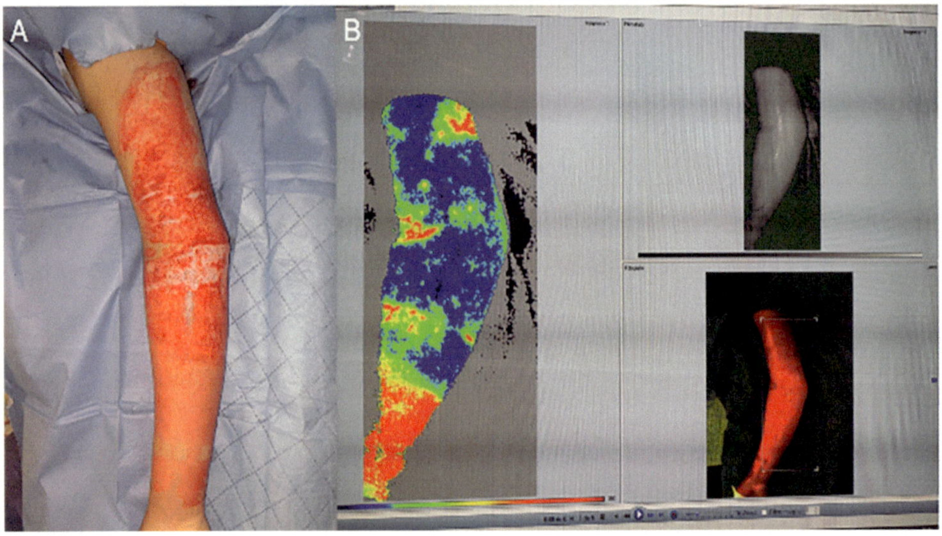

Figure 2.
Assessment of burn depth using Doppler ultrasound.

For NexoBrid® to work optimally, the target burned surfaces—deep-partial-thickness (grade IIB) and even full-thickness (grade III) injuries—must first be adequately hydrated. No silver-sulfadiazine creams or povidone-iodine (Betadine®) dressings should be applied beforehand, as these agents can inactivate the enzyme complex.

Immediately before NexoBrid® application, the wound is thoroughly irrigated to remove blisters, soot, foreign particles, and any loose devitalised tissue. Lavage is performed with sterile isotonic 0.9% sodium-chloride solution and Prontosan® (B. Braun, Germany). Use of Prontosan—both before and after the enzymatic phase—is strongly recommended, because its polyhexanide-based surfactant both cleanses the wound bed and minimises microbial burden without impairing bromelain activity (**Figure 3**).

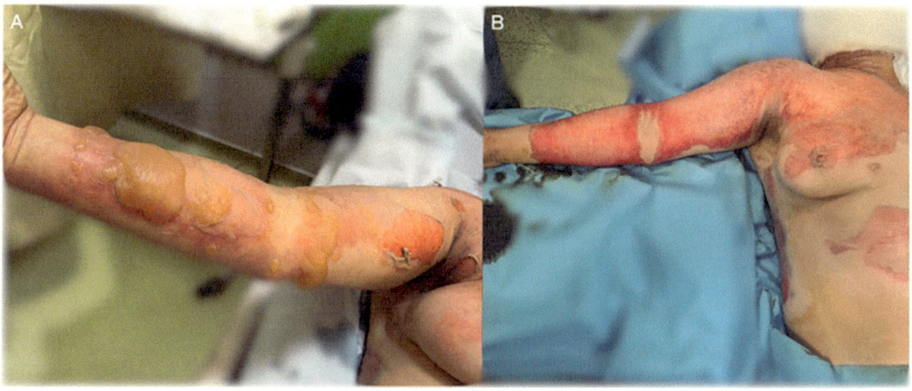

Figure 3.
Burn of the upper limb. (A) Before wound irrigation and (B) after irrigation with removal of blisters and devitalised tissue.

Hydrogel dressings may also be applied to hydrate and condition the burned integument before enzymatic debridement; a minimum pre-hydration interval of 2 hours is recommended. Adequate analgesia is mandatory both during and after NexoBrid® application. Clinical studies suggest maintaining pain control for at least 48 hours post-debridement, with extension as required according to burn depth, extent, and each patient's individual pain threshold.

With respect to anaesthetic choice for enzymatic debridement in burn patients, loco-regional techniques are preferred whenever the anatomical site permits, thereby avoiding general anaesthesia with endotracheal intubation. When NexoBrid® is applied to the upper limb, an axillary, infraclavicular, supraclavicular, or interscalene block is selected according to the exact level of injury. For lower-extremity burns, femoral or sciatic nerve blocks are favoured. Any of these regional approaches may be supplemented with intravenous sedation. Burns of the head, neck, thorax, or upper abdomen, by contrast, necessitate general anaesthesia with endotracheal intubation. To maintain adequate analgesia for at least 48 hours after NexoBrid® application, a continuous-infusion catheter delivering a long-acting local anaesthetic is recommended.

2. *Isolation of the burn from adjacent healthy skin.* Surrounding intact skin is protected with gauze dressings thoroughly impregnated with petroleum jelly—or a comparable greasy ointment—and firmly anchored in place. Any prior escharotomy incisions are shielded in the same fashion. When NexoBrid® is applied to facial burns, the eyes must be covered with a double-layer compress (**Figure 4**).

3. *Preparation and application of the product*. Reconstitute NexoBrid® by gradually mixing the lyophilised powder into the gel, then spread the resulting suspension with a spatula in a uniform layer 1.5–3 mm thick, exactly as specified by the manufacturer (**Figure 5**).

4. *Cover and seal the treated area with a non-absorbent film*, then add a second layer: Either sterile gauze compresses or an additional hydrofilm sheet: To secure the dressing (**Figure 6**)

5. *The bromelain-based formulation is left in situ for 4 hours*; after this dwell time, the agent is rinsed away with sterile saline and Prontosan®, using gauze pads,

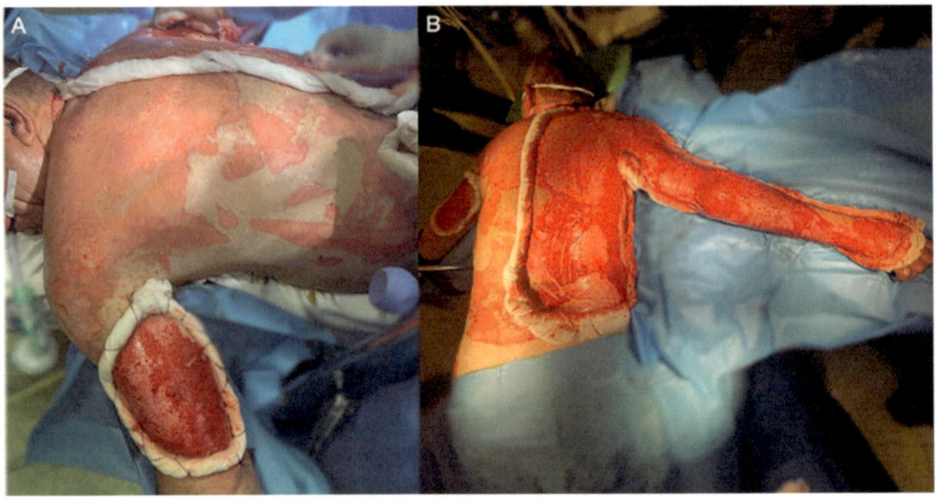

Figure 4.
Barrier isolation of the target debridement field from adjacent uninvolved integument.

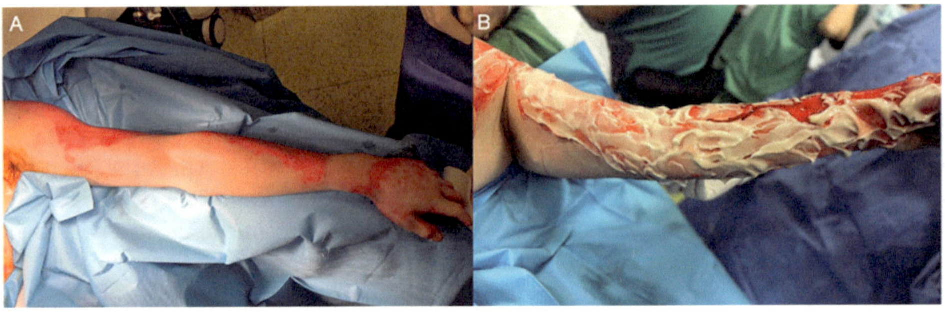

Figure 5.
(A) Circumferential deep-partial (II-B degree) and full-thickness (III-rd degree) burn of the upper limb; (B) topical enzymatic debridement with NexoBrid®.

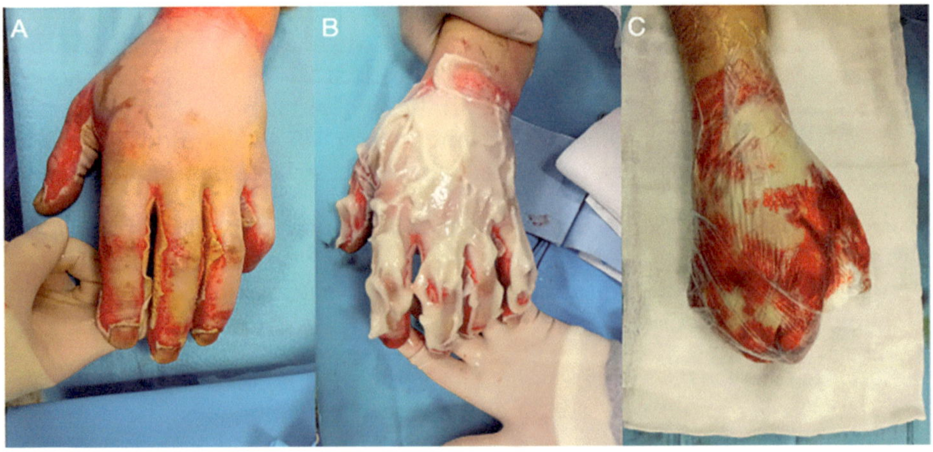

Figure 6.
(A) Deep burn on the dorsal aspect of the hand; (B) application of NexoBrid® to the dorsal hand burn; (C) treated area sealed with an occlusive dressing for 4 hours.

spatulas, or mildly abrasive sponges to remove both the residual preparation and the loosened eschar. A hydrosurgery system can also be employed to complete the debridement (**Figure 7**).

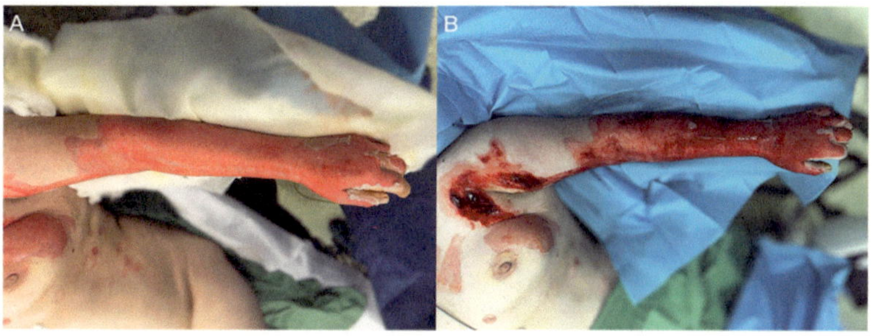

Figure 7.
(A) Circumferential burn of the left forearm and (B) appearance after removal of the debriding agent and irrigation with Prontosan® (B. Braun, Melsungen, Germany).

6. *Prontosan® (B. Braun, Melsungen, Germany) dressings.*

7. *The debrided area must be covered to prevent desiccation*, the formation of pseudo-eschar, and infection by applying a permanent or temporary skin substitute, such as Suprathel®, Biobrane®, or Mepitel®, or allografts in cases of burn wounds showing vital dermis and good healing potential or autografts in deep burns requiring surgical treatment (**Figures 8** and **9**) [30, 51, 56–58].

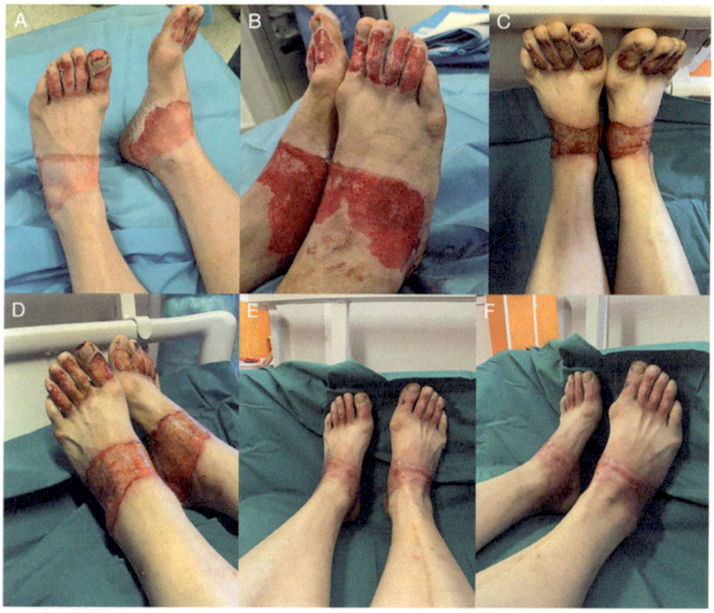

Figure 8.
Enzymatic debridement sequence: (A) burn wound after initial lavage; (B) right leg immediately post-debridement; (C) application of the enzymatic agent to the left leg; (D) wound appearance 3 days post-debridement; (E) wound appearance 6 days post-debridement; (F) spontaneous healing outcome following enzymatic debridement.

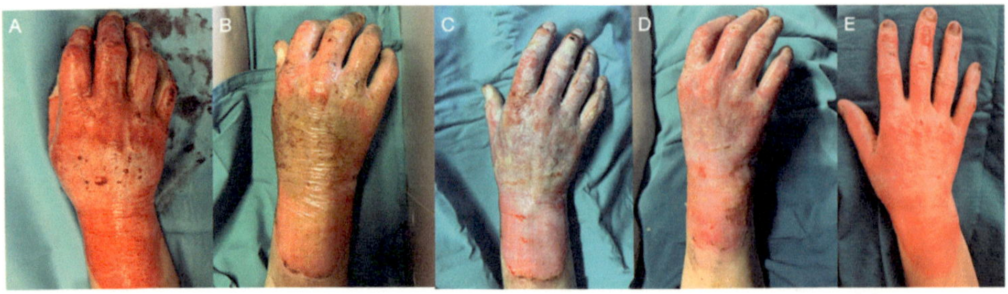

Figure 9.
Evolution of a grade II-B burn on the dorsal right hand following enzymatic debridement: (A) immediate post-debridement appearance; (B) wound aspect at 4 days post-debridement; (C) wound aspect at 10 days post-debridement; (D) wound aspect at 14 days post-debridement; (E) complete healing achieved by directed epithelialisation.

8. *Assessment 24: 48 hours after debridement*, the observed effects, and the ensuing therapeutic plan for the residual wound: Either spontaneous healing through directed epithelialisation, subsequently supported by topical agents or skin coverage by one of several grafting methods conventional split-thickness skin grafting harvested with an electric dermatome or meek micrografting (**Figures 10** and **11**)

A schematic outline of the steps for employing NXB is shown in **Figure 12**.

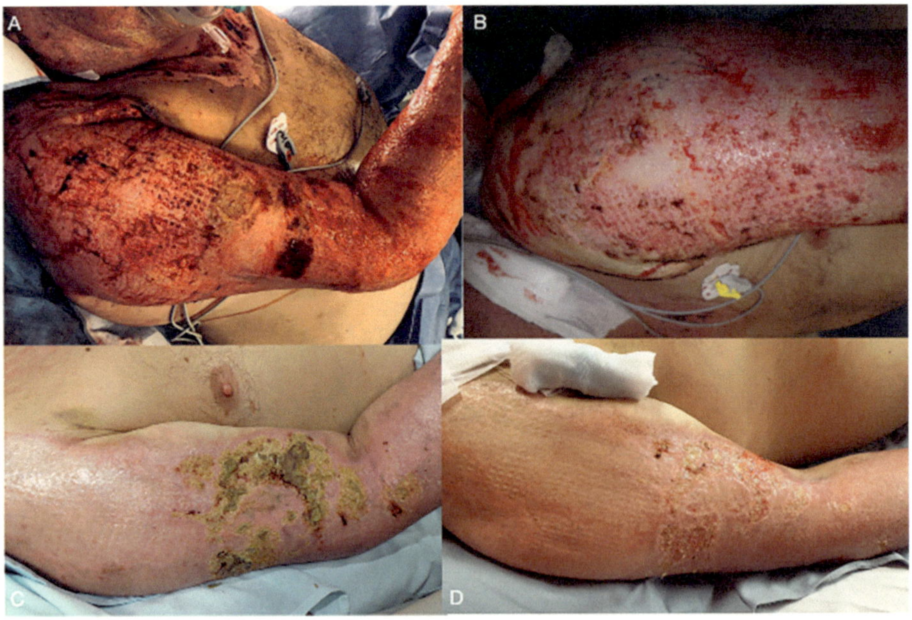

Figure 10.
(A) Post-burn regions enzymatically debrided and covered with Meek micrografts at the shoulder and upper arm; (B) healing in progress; (C, D) spontaneous epithelialisation of the forearm and complete integration with healed burn areas at the shoulder and proximal third of the arm.

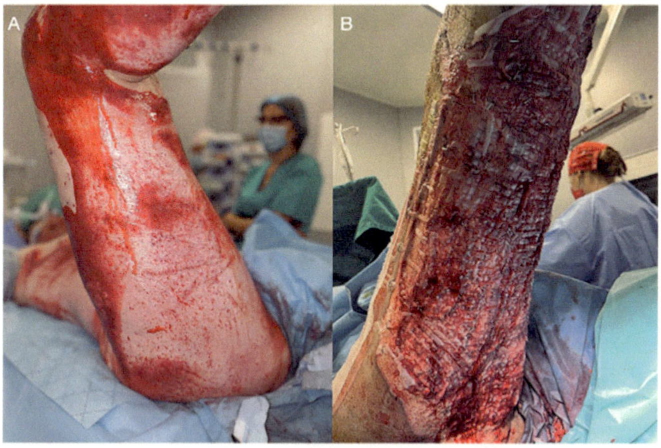

Figure 11.
(A) Post-enzymatic debridement appearance of a circumferential burn on the right lower limb and (B) coverage of the initially enzymatically debrided areas with Meek micrografts.

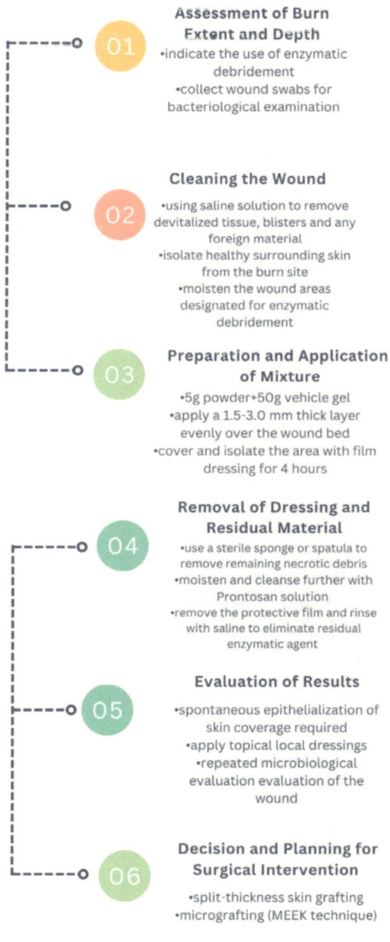

Figure 12.
The steps for employing NXB.

4. Use of enzymatic debridement in special anatomical regions: The face and the hand

4.1 Use of NexoBrid® on the face

Although initially regarded with caution, enzymatic debridement has progressively gained acceptance for use on the face, as growing clinical evidence has confirmed its safety and efficacy. Facial burns affect up to 5.3% of all burn patients and even small lesions can inflict major aesthetic and psychosocial harm [9]. Beyond visible scarring, functional sequelae involving the eyelids, nasal alae, lips, and oral commissures can profoundly compromise daily activities. Because facial skin is thin and highly vascularised, timely debridement that preserves the maximum amount of viable tissue accelerates healing and improves the final cosmetic outcome [9].

The 2020 update of the European consensus on bromelain-based enzymatic debridement specifically addressed deep facial burns, emphasising that safe application of NexoBrid® hinges on meticulous protection of natural orifices—particularly the eyes—through careful shielding and moisture control [30].

Reports in the literature outline several techniques for protecting the eyes during facial application of NexoBrid®. Schulz et al. describe covering the eyes with Bepanthen® ointment (Bayer, Germany), sealing them beneath an occlusive plaster, and then surrounding the area with a ring of Adapt® paste (Hollister, Germany) [9]. Ferancikova et al. achieved similar protection of the orbital region—and of the external auditory canal—using a generous layer of sterile [59], medical-grade petroleum jelly (**Figures 13** and **14**).

Due to the need for complex and reliable ocular protection methods, enzymatic debridement is difficult to apply in cases of eyelid burns, where there is a significant risk of ocular damage. Given the extreme thinness of the eyelid skin, intermediate and deep burns which are the typical indications for enzymatic debridement often lead to exposure of the tarsal plate. In such situations, the use of enzymatic agents may be of limited benefit, as the risk to the eye outweighs the expected therapeutic advantage.

A similar issue arises with the use of NexoBrid® in burns affecting the auricular pavilion. However, enzymatic debridement may be more feasible in this location, as the external auditory canal can be easily and safely protected during the procedure.

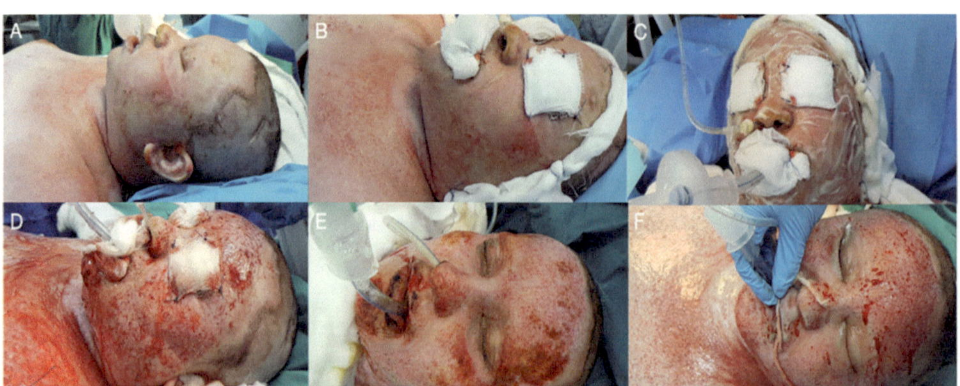

Figure 13.
(A) Full-thickness burn involving the face and anterior thorax; (B) isolation of zones prepared for enzymatic debridement; (C) application of the enzymatic debridement agent; (D) appearance of debrided areas immediately after NXB removal; (E) removal of protective eye and periocular dressings, confirming intact adjacent skin; (F) debrided facial region 24 hours after enzymatic debridement.

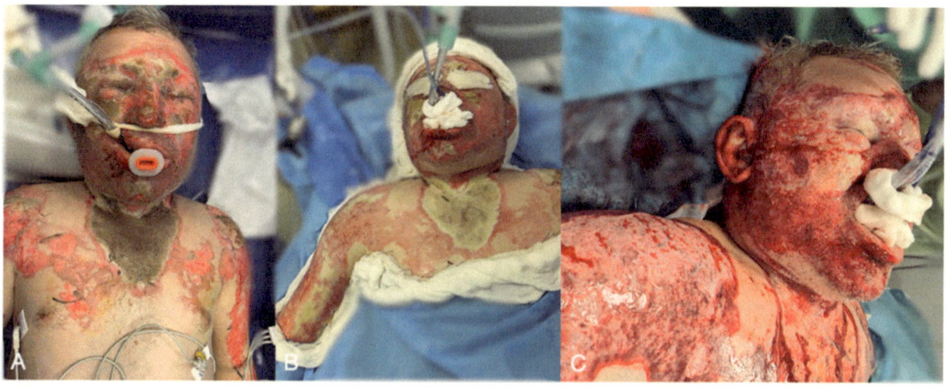

Figure 14.
(A) Full-thickness (grade III) facial burn; (B) enzymatically debrided burn at 5 days post-debridement, showing active epithelialisation; (C) outcome at 3 weeks post-debridement – areas fully or partially re-epithelialised, with cicatricial ectropion of the left eye.

4.2 Use of enzymatic debridement on the hands

Burns of the hand can result in profound aesthetic and functional deficits. Treating such injuries is particularly challenging: the hand is a highly complex organ whose fine motor capabilities and appearance—alongside the face—form our primary interface with the outside world, underpinning interpersonal interaction and carrying powerful symbolic meaning [60–65]. For this reason, every hand-burn case must be managed with the overarching objectives of preserving anatomical integrity and function while minimising scarring, thereby limiting any long-term impact on the patient's social, professional, and personal life [63].

Because the dorsal skin of the hand is exceptionally thin, medium- and deep-depth burns often leave extensor tendons exposed. In these circumstances, simple coverage with a split-thickness skin graft is not feasible, and alternative reconstructive strategies must be pursued [60–65]. Frequently, the lack of healthy adjacent tissue necessitates distant flap techniques, which entail extensive surgery, produce additional scars, and carry the added morbidity of donor sites [65].

Accordingly, the optimal strategy is a highly selective debridement technique that preserves every viable island of intact skin (**Figure 15**).

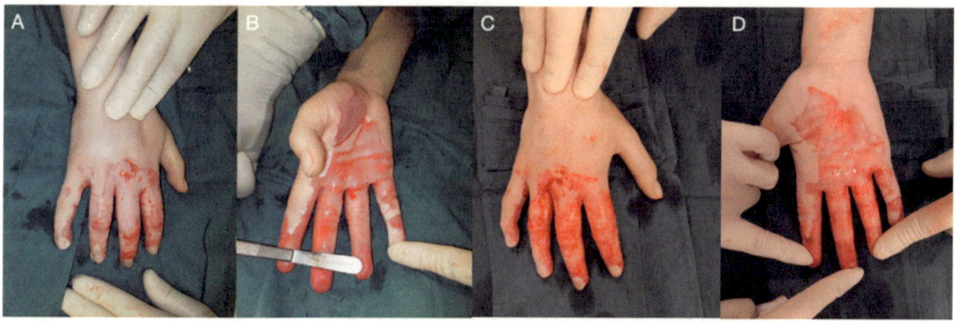

Figure 15.
(A, B) Deep burn from prolonged contact with wax and (C, D) appearance after enzymatic debridement.

NexoBrid® is now regarded as the first-line treatment for hand burns, because it removes only necrotic tissue while sparing every viable skin island—sources of epithelial cells that drive directed re-epithelialisation and later wound closure. Although surgical excision followed by grafting is still the classic standard for medium- and full-thickness burns elsewhere, for deep-partial and full-thickness burns of the hand the preferred standard is selective enzymatic debridement, with grafting reserved for cases in which residual dermal cover proves insufficient [60–65].

Selective enzymatic debridement followed by directed epithelialisation permits continuous mobilisation of the hands throughout the healing phase, so that functional sequelae are minimal or altogether absent [64].

By contrast, split-thickness skin grafts on the hand require a postoperative period of immobilisation to secure graft take, with an attendant risk of stiffness and contracture [61–64]. In addition, spontaneous healing after enzymatic debridement consistently delivers superior aesthetic outcomes: the resulting scars are thinner, more pliable, and better colour-matched than those produced by conventional grafting (**Figure 16**) [61–65].

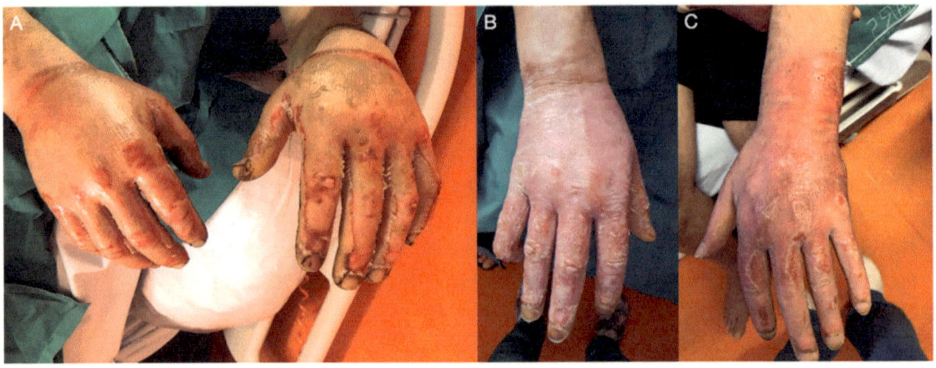

Figure 16.
Burn of dorsal faces of both hands: (A) Day 2 post-debridement, (B, C) complete epithelialisation.

The effectiveness of enzymatic debridement on the hands must also be evaluated in relation to the numerous flexion creases present at the level of the fingers, both dorsally and palmarly, as well as at the wrist.

These anatomical areas are particularly challenging to cover using split-thickness skin grafts, as graft contraction frequently occurs, leading to significant functional impairment. In such cases, outcomes are often inferior to those achieved through directed epithelialisation. This principle applies to all areas with flexion folds—including the elbow, knee, ankle, neck, and others.

In paediatric patients, enzymatic debridement is notably more effective when applied to the hands and other flexural regions compared to adults. This is due to the significant advantage of avoiding skin grafting in children, as skin grafts do not grow proportionally with the child. As a result, repeated grafting procedures may be necessary throughout childhood until growth is complete.

4.3 Use of enzymatic debridement in the prevention and management of compartment syndrome arising from circumferential limb burns

Compartment syndrome occurs when intra-compartmental pressure exceeds the perfusion pressure of the blood vessels within that compartment, ultimately resulting in tissue ischaemia and necrosis. It is a surgical emergency. Although there are multiple etiologies, the most common triggers of compartment syndrome are traumatic injuries and burns [66].

In burn injuries, compartment syndrome more frequently develops in the limbs when the burns are circumferential and of deep thickness. In these cases, the pathogenesis may involve interstitial fluid accumulation that raises intra-compartmental pressure or the inelastic burned skin acting like a tourniquet, likewise increasing compartmental pressure [66].

To prevent irreversible muscle contracture, nerve damage, and ultimately tissue necrosis with potential limb loss, emergent fasciotomies are indicated [66, 67].

Fasciotomies constitute a surgical intervention associated with inherent risks, including significant blood loss. With the advent of enzymatic debridement, in cases of early circular limb burns—within the first hours post-injury—the onset or even treatment of compartment syndrome can be managed using NexoBrid®. The primary concern, however, is the four-hour action window of NXB's proteolytic enzymes, during which there is effectively no real-time control over the evolution of compartment pressures [67, 68].

Nevertheless, studies have demonstrated that enzymatic debridement is effective in preventing, managing, and treating compartment syndrome in deep circumferential burns (**Figure 17**).

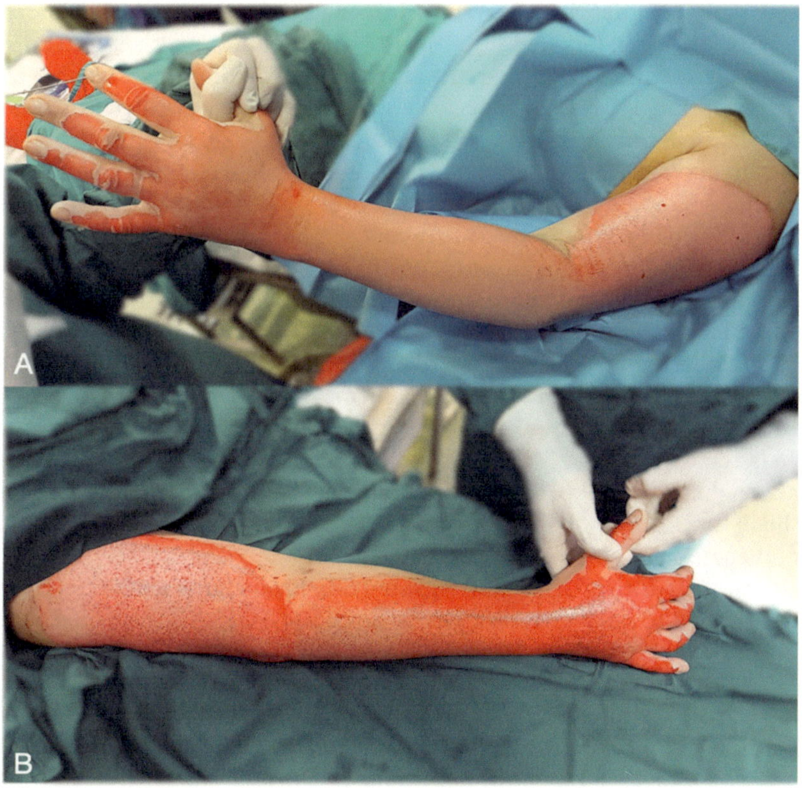

Figure 17.
Deep circumferential burn of the forearm: (A) immediate post-burn aspect and (B) immediate post-debridement aspect.

European consensus guidelines indicate that early eschar removal with NexoBrid® can reliably prevent the need for surgical escharotomy of the upper extremities [30, 53]. By excising the eschar, one averts the development of elevated pressures within the subcutaneous and subfascial compartments; performing this intervention promptly also attenuates local inflammation and oedema, both of which drive burn-related compartment syndrome [30].

Enzymatic debridement with a bromelain-based preparation (NXB) is a safe, feasible, and effective method for performing an "enzymatic escharotomy" to counteract compartment-pressure build-up in deep extremity burns and thereby reduce the need for surgical escharotomy [66, 67].

This enzymatic escharotomy must, of course, be performed early. In cases of very deep or extensive burns (exceeding 50% TBSA), it may still be necessary to combine enzymatic debridement with a conventional surgical escharotomy [67].

The literature reports shorter hospital stays and fewer surgical interventions in patients who underwent enzymatic debridement to prevent burn-induced compartment syndrome. As with other burn wounds, enzymatic debridement is then followed either by spontaneous re-epithelialisation or by coverage of denuded areas using split-thickness skin grafts harvested with an electric dermatome or by Meek micrografting [30, 66, 67].

5. Discussion

The high global incidence of burn injuries—and the resulting annual mortality exceeding 180,000—renders these traumas a critical public health concern [69, 70]. This heightened attention has driven the search for novel therapies, leading to the widespread adoption of bromelain-based enzymatic debridement (NexoBrid®) as a primary modality in burn care worldwide [30].

Bromelain, derived from pineapple, was first described in 1891 by Venezuelan scientist Vicente Marcano, with its extraction process developed 3 years later [71]. It is a mixture of proteolytic enzymes—primarily comosain and ananain—that catalyse the breakdown of proteins into amino acids. Beyond its role in wound debridement, bromelain is employed in the treatment of various ENT, respiratory, cardiovascular, and rheumatologic conditions [72].

Bromelain is extracted as a glycosylated monomeric protein, found in both the stem and the fruit of pineapple. The two isoforms—stem bromelain and fruit bromelain—are highly homologous, differing primarily in their isoelectric points: stem bromelain is alkaline (pH > 9.5), while fruit bromelain is acidic (pH ≈ 4.6). Their molecular weights, optimal pH, and temperature ranges are very similar. The key differences lie in their amino-acid sequences, which confer subtle variations in substrate affinity and enzymatic kinetics [71].

In addition to its anti-inflammatory properties, bromelain's antibacterial activity has been attributed to its constituent phytochemicals—tannins, saponins, and flavonoids. Ali et al. have demonstrated that bromelain inhibits the growth of *Escherichia coli* and *Proteus* species [73, 74].

Potential adverse effects of this enzymatic compound have also been investigated. Animal studies (in rabbits and mice) have shown that bromelain exhibits very low toxicity, even at high doses, without detectable impairment of cardiac, renal, or gastrointestinal function, nor significant alterations in haematologic parameters [51].

The use of the bromelain-based compound—NexoBrid®—for burn debridement has expanded dramatically worldwide in recent years. Consequently, multiple studies have evaluated NXB in burn therapy, and both national and European consensus guidelines have been developed to standardise its application (**Table 1**).

Countries such as Spain, Italy, Poland and Romania, have issued and published national consensus statements on NXB use, all of which align with and adhere to the two European consensus documents from 2018 and 2020 (**Table 2**) [30, 53, 75–80].

In Spain, in 2017, Martinez Mendez published a national consensus on NXB use that involved seven burn units across the country [75].

In 2023, Serracanta et al. updated this earlier consensus by including not only plastic surgeons but also intensivists and anesthesiologists—16 experts in total. Of the nine certified burn centres in Spain, eight participated in the 2023 consensus.

Region.	Author/ year	Panellists	Patients	Evaluated topics	Key contributions
Europe	Hirche C et al. [53]	Austria, Belgium, Germany, Italy, Slovak Republic, Spain, Switzerland, the United Kingdom	500	• Indications • Pain management • Anaesthesia- Timing and technique of application • Post-intervention wound care • Skin grafting after ED • Blood loss • Cost-effectiveness • Training & learning curve • Research needs	• ED indicated for hands, feet, face • Not for chemical burns • Suitable for thermal, scald, flame, contact burns • Safe up to 15% TBSA/ session (up to 30% off-label) • Regional anaesthesia recommended for limbs • Late application = >72 h • Eschar removal within 7 days • Reapplication not recommended after failure
Europe	Hirche C et al. [30]	Austria, Belgium, Germany, Italy, Norway, Poland, Romania, Spain, Switzerland, the United Kingdom	1232	• Indications • Pain & anaesthesia • Large surface use • Timing • Post-debridement wound care • Grafting • Scar & revision • Cost-efficiency • Patient perspective • Logistics • Training	• Application timing: immediate (<12 h), early (12–72 h), delayed (>72 h) • No use in chemical burns • Suitable for full-thickness burns • Early use may prevent compartment syndrome • Highly recommended for facial, hand, foot, perineal, genital burns • Up to 15% TBSA/session sequentially • Local anaesthesia useful in minor burns

ED – enzymatic debridement, TBSA – total burn surface area, h – hour.

Table 1.
European consensus guidelines on the use of NexoBrid® in burn care.

Country	Author/year	Panellists	Patients	Evaluated topics	Key contributions
Spain	Martinez-Mendez et al. [75]	Burn units of: Madrid, Barcelona, Zaragoza, Valencia, A Coruña, Murcia, Valladolid	350	Indications, recommendations	• ED indicated for deep dermal burns • Limited experience with electrical burns • Use up to 15% TBSA • Limited experience on the face • Reapplication protocol not defined • Avoids escharotomy in circular burns
Spain	Serracanta J. et al. [76]	Burn units of: Barcelona, Madrid, Zaragoza, Valencia, A Coruña, Bizkaia, Seville, Valladolid	>1000 cases	Indications, critical patients, pain, application, post-ED care	• ED indicated for deep dermal burns • Used by experienced professionals only • Off-label for paediatric patients • Effective on face, hands, neck, neckline • Safe on up to 15% TBSA • Not for chemical/high-voltage burns • Avoids surgical escharotomy in circumferential burns
Spain	Gonzalez et al. [77]	Burn units of: Barcelona, Madrid, Zaragoza, Valencia, A Coruña, Vizcaya, Seville, Valladolid, Alicante	Approx. 1500 cases	Admission, pain control, application/ removal, post-ED	• Trained nurses manage ED patients • Plastic surgeon provides education • Better scar quality and fewer sequelae • Optimising wound bed for healing or grafting

Country	Author/year	Panellists	Patients	Evaluated topics	Key contributions
Italy	Ranno R et al. [78]	Burn centres of: Catania, Bari, Brindisi, Cesena, Genova, Milano, Napoli, Palermo, Parma, Pisa, Roma, Sassari, Torino, Verona	1068	Indications, pain, timing, technique, post-ED, mass casualty	• Not for epidermal/superficial burns • Requires trained staff • Useful on face, hands, neck, décolleté • Reduces bleeding on the chest/abdomen • Max 15% TBSA per application • Reapplication possible >24 h • Not for chemical/electrical burns • Useful in eschar removal from circumferential burns
Poland	Korzeniowski et al. [79]	Burn centres of: Cracow, Gryfice, Siemianowice Śląskie, Poznań, Łęczna	>500 cases	Indications, pain, anaesthesia, large surfaces, timing, prep, post-ED, outcomes, cost, training	• Recommended for deep dermal/full-thickness burns • Safe with an experienced team • Not for chemical/electrical burns • Effective for hands, face, groin • Max 15% TBSA/session • Indicated for circumferential burns • -Pain management needed • Delayed use (>72 h) still possible

Country	Author/year	Panellists	Patients	Evaluated topics	Key contributions
Romania	Marinescu S. et al. [80]	7 healthcare units	342	Indications, surface, prep, timing, pain, anaesthesia, post-ED, grafting, follow-up, patient view, logistics, training	• Use within 24 h • Face, hands, feet burns (max 15% TBSA) • Indicated for thermal burns (not chemical/electrical) • Reduces need for escharotomy in circumferential burns • Facial/genital/perineal burns highly indicated • Limb burns managed with loco-regional anaesthesia

ED- enzymatic debridement, prep – preparation, TBSA – total burn surface area, h-hour.

Table 2.
National consensus guidelines on the use of NexoBrid® in burn care.

As with other guidelines, this document was aligned with the Summary of Product Characteristics (SPC) [76].

In Italy, Ranno R et al. reported a consensus on NXB use in 2021, led by two principal investigators and encompassing 20 experts from 14 burn centres nationwide [78].

In Poland, a 2022 consensus was developed with input from five burn centres. In Romania, Marinescu et al. published the 2020 consensus, which included experts from four health units [79, 80].

Both national and European consensus guidelines were developed according to the Oxford Level of Evidence Classification System. The inaugural European consensus convened panellists from Austria, Belgium, Germany, Italy, the Slovak Republic, Spain, Switzerland, and the United Kingdom. This consensus examined multiple facets of enzymatic debridement in burn care, including: the indications for enzymatic debridement; pain management and choice of anaesthetic technique; the optimal timing of application; precise application methodology; post-debridement wound care; the timing of skin grafting; dosing and haemorrhage control; and, critically, the economic impact, requisite training protocols, and associated learning curve [53]. Since the 2017 consensus, NexoBrid® has been recognised as both effective and indicated for burns of the hands, feet, and face [53]. The second European consensus on enzymatic debridement included expert panels from Austria, Belgium, Germany, Italy, Norway, Poland, Romania, Spain, Switzerland, and the United Kingdom. While many topics mirrored those of the inaugural consensus, this update also incorporated: rigorous evaluation of clinical outcomes following enzymatic debridement; standardised protocols for scar management and revision; formal cost-effectiveness analyses; the integration of patient-reported perspectives; and detailed considerations of NexoBrid® logistics and supply-chain requirements [30]. In the second European consensus, precise definitions were established for the temporal categories "very early," "early," and "late," corresponding to post-burn intervals of <12 hours, 12–72 hours, and > 72 hours, respectively [30]. A pivotal advancement was the formal introduction of the "enzymatic escharotomy" concept, defined as the application of enzymatic debridement within the first 12 hours after injury in cases of circumferential burns; this approach can both prevent the development of compartment syndrome and treat incipient syndrome without resorting to surgical decompression incisions [66].

Application of enzymatic debridement for burns covering less than 2% TBSA is generally not recommended, primarily for cost-efficiency reasons. Regarding anaesthetic technique, small treatment areas may be managed under local anaesthesia; limb burns typically employ regional blocks; and spinal anaesthesia is also an option. As a broad recommendation, procedural sedation and analgesia are preferred over general anaesthesia with endotracheal intubation [81, 82].

The indications for NexoBrid® encompass both intermediate- and full-thickness burns. Reapplication to the same area—when initial debridement fails to achieve the desired effect—is generally not recommended and is permissible only in exceptional cases. The consensus emphasises enzymatic debridement for burns of the hands, feet, perineal, and genital regions; for facial burns, ED is both indicated and efficacious, provided that meticulous protection of the eyes and natural orifices is maintained. Preparation protocols and timing remain identical to those defined in the first European consensus, including the limit of 15% TBSA per application.

Prior to NXB application, any pre-existing or burn-induced coagulopathies must be corrected to ensure patient safety. If no spontaneous epithelialisation is evident 21 days post-debridement, surgical skin grafting should be considered [83]. Recent updates have extended NXB indications to paediatric patients: children aged

4–18 years may be treated on up to 15% TBSA in a single session, while in those aged 0–3 years the maximum is 10% TBSA.

In light of these advances, Romania is preparing to revise its national consensus on enzymatic debridement, drawing on the collective experience of six medical centres using NXB.

6. Conclusions

Enzymatic debridement offers a valuable alternative to surgical excision, providing advantages in terms of speed, tissue selectivity, and overall safety. Bromelain-based debridement, particularly with NexoBrid®, has shown superior capacity to preserve viable tissue, minimise blood loss typically associated with surgical excision, and reduce the need for skin graft donor sites. These benefits are linked to lower morbidity, improved functional outcomes, and earlier patient mobilisation. Additionally, scars resulting from enzymatic debridement tend to have a more favourable aesthetic appearance compared to those following surgical treatment.

However, while current findings are promising, further large-scale studies are required to conclusively establish the safety, efficacy, and appropriate clinical indications of bromelain-based therapy. At present, surgical debridement followed by autografting remains the gold standard in burn management. Nonetheless, combining enzymatic and surgical approaches may be beneficial in treating extensive burns of varying depth.

The effectiveness of enzymatic debridement in chemical and electrical burns, as well as its safety in cases involving larger TBSA involvement, remains to be fully clarified. Notably, our observations suggest that early application of NexoBrid® in deep, circumferential limb burns may help prevent the onset of compartment syndrome—though this hypothesis warrants further investigation.

Conflict of interest

The authors declare no conflict of interest.

Acronyms and abbreviations

NXB	Nexobrid®
ED	enzymatic debridement
TBSA	total burn surface area
SPC	Summary of Product Characteristics

Author details

Mihaela Pertea[1,2]

1 Grigore T Popa University of Medicine and Pharmacy, Iasi, Romania

2 Plastic Surgery and Reconstructive Microsurgery Department and Burn Unit, Sf Spiridon Emergency County Hospital, Iasi, Romania

*Address all correspondence to: mihaela.pertea@umfiasi.ro

References

[1] Siegwart LC, Böcker AH, Diehm YF, Kotsougiani-Fischer D, Erdmann S, Ziegler B, et al. Enzymatic debridement for burn wound care: Interrater reliability and impact of experience in post-intervention therapy decision. Journal of Burn Care & Research. 2021;**42**(5):953-961. DOI: 10.1093/jbcr/iraa218

[2] Hofmaenner DA, Steiger P, Schuepbach RA, Klinzing S, Waldner M, Klein H, et al. Safety of enzymatic debridement in extensive burns larger than 15% total body surface area. Burns. 2021;**47**(4):796-804. DOI: 10.1016/j.burns.2020.10.012

[3] Atiyeh B, Makkawi K, Beaineh P. Burn wounds and enzymatic debridement (ED)-past, present, and future. Journal of Burn Care & Research. 2024;**45**(4):864-876. DOI: 10.1093/jbcr/irae059

[4] Kakagia DD, Karadimas EJ. The efficacy of versajet™ hydrosurgery system in burn surgery. A systematic review. Journal of Burn Care & Research. 2018;**39**(2):188-200. DOI: 10.1097/BCR.0000000000000561

[5] Kwa KAA, Goei H, Breederveld RS, Middelkoop E, van der Vlies CH, van Baar ME. A systematic review on surgical and nonsurgical debridement techniques of burn wounds. Journal of Plastic, Reconstructive & Aesthetic Surgery. 2019;**72**(11):1752-1762. DOI: 10.1016/j.bjps.2019.07.006

[6] De Decker I, De Graeve L, Hoeksema H, Monstrey S, Verbelen J, De Coninck P, et al. Enzymatic debridement: Past, present, and future. Acta Chirurgica Belgica. 2022;**122**(4):279-295. DOI: 10.1080/00015458.2022.2068746

[7] Shoham Y, Shapira E, Haik J, Harats M, Egozi D, Robinson D, et al. Bromelain-based enzymatic debridement of chronic wounds: Results of a multicentre randomized controlled trial. Wound Repair and Regeneration. 2021;**29**(6):899-907. DOI: 10.1111/wrr.12958

[8] Manna B, Nahirniak P, Morrison CA. Wound Debridement. In: StatPearls. Treasure Island (FL): StatPearls Publishing; 2025

[9] Schulz A, Fuchs PC, Rothermundt I, Hoffmann A, Rosenberg L, Shoham Y, et al. Enzymatic debridement of deeply burned faces: Healing and early scarring based on tissue preservation compared to traditional surgical debridement. Burns. 2017;**43**(6):1233-1243. DOI: 10.1016/j.burns.2017.02.016

[10] Snyder RJ, Fife C, Moore Z. Components and quality measures of DIME (devitalized tissue, infection/inflammation, moisture balance, and edge preparation) in wound care. Advances in Skin & Wound Care. 2016;**29**(5):205-215. DOI: 10.1097/01.ASW.0000482354.01988.b

[11] Kirshen C, Woo K, Ayello EA, Sibbald RG. Debridement: A vital component of wound bed preparation. Advances in Skin & Wound Care. 2006;**19**(9):506-517. quiz 517-9. DOI: 10.1097/00129334-200611000-00011

[12] Thomas DC, Tsu CL, Nain RA, Arsat N, Fun SS, Lah NASN. The role of debridement in wound bed preparation in chronic wound: A narrative review. Annals of Medicine and Surgery (London). 2021;**71**:102876. DOI: 10.1016/j.amsu.2021.102876

[13] Kamolz LP, Wild T. Wound bed preparation: The impact of debridement and wound cleansing. Wound Medicine. 2013;**1**:44-50

[14] Ramundo J, Gray M. Enzymatic wound debridement. Journal of Wound, Ostomy, and Continence Nursing. 2008;**35**(3):273-280. DOI: 10.1097/01.WON.0000319125.21854.78

[15] Kwa KAA, van Haasterecht L, Elgersma A, Breederveld RS, Groot ML, van Zuijlen PPM, et al. Effective enzymatic debridement of burn wounds depends on the denaturation status of collagen. Wound Repair and Regeneration. 2020;**28**(5):666-675. DOI: 10.1111/wrr.12827

[16] Mayer DO, Tettelbach WH, Ciprandi G, Downie F, Hampton J, Hodgson H, et al. Best practice for wound debridement. Journal of Wound Care. 2024;**33**(Sup6b):S1-S32. DOI: 10.12968/jowc.2024.33.Sup6b.S1

[17] Choo J, Nixon J, Nelson A, McGinnis E. Autolytic debridement for pressure ulcers. Cochrane Database of Systematic Reviews. 2019;**2019**(6):CD011331. DOI: 10.1002/14651858.CD011331.pub2

[18] Turkmen A, Graham K, McGrouther DA. Therapeutic applications of the larvae for wound debridement. Journal of Plastic, Reconstructive & Aesthetic Surgery. 2010;**63**(1):184-188. DOI: 10.1016/j.bjps.2008.08.070

[19] Eriksson E, Liu PY, Schultz GS, Martins-Green MM, Tanaka R, Weir D, et al. Chronic wounds: Treatment consensus. Wound Repair and Regeneration. 2022;**30**(2):156-171. DOI: 10.1111/wrr.12994. Epub 2022 Feb 7. Erratum in: Wound Repair Regen. 2022 Jul;30(4):536. DOI: 10.1111/wrr.13035

[20] Nowak M, Mehrholz D, Barańska-Rybak W, Nowicki RJ. Wound debridement products and techniques: Clinical examples and literature review. Postepy Dermatologii I Alergologii. 2022;**39**(3):479-490. DOI: 10.5114/ada.2022.117572

[21] Whitaker IS, Twine C, Whitaker MJ, Welck M, Brown CS, Shandall A. Larval therapy from antiquity to the present day: Mechanisms of action, clinical applications and future potential. Postgraduate Medical Journal. 2007;**83**(980):409-413. DOI: 10.1136/pgmj.2006.055905

[22] Greene E, Avsar P, Moore Z, Nugent L, O'Connor T, Patton D. What is the effect of larval therapy on the debridement of venous leg ulcers? A systematic review. Journal of Tissue Viability. 2021;**30**(3):301-309. DOI: 10.1016/j.jtv.2021.05.005

[23] Lam T, Beraja GE, Lev-Tov H. Efficacy of larval therapy for wounds: A systematic review and meta-analysis. Journal of Clinical Medicine. 2025;**14**(2):315. DOI: 10.3390/jcm14020315

[24] Diefenbeck M, Haustedt N, Schmidt HG. Surgical debridement to optimise wound conditions and healing. International Wound Journal. 2013;**10**(Suppl. 1):43-47. DOI: 10.1111/iwj.12187

[25] Smith F, Dryburgh N, Donaldson J, Mitchell M. Debridement for surgical wounds. Cochrane Database of Systematic Reviews. 2013;**2013**(9):CD006214. DOI: 10.1002/14651858.CD006214.pub4. Update in: Cochrane Database Syst Rev. 2024 May 7;5:CD006214. DOI: 10.1002/14651858.CD006214.pub5

[26] Heitzmann W, Fuchs PC, Schiefer JL. Historical perspectives on

the development of current standards of care for enzymatic debridement. Medicina (Kaunas, Lithuania). 2020;**56**(12):706. DOI: 10.3390/medicina56120706

[27] Bernagozzi F, Orlandi C, Purpura V, Morselli PG, Melandri D. The enzymatic debridement for the treatment of burns of indeterminate depth. Journal of Burn Care & Research. 2020;**41**(5):1084-1091. DOI: 10.1093/jbcr/iraa051

[28] Cordts T, Horter J, Vogelpohl J, Kremer T, Kneser U, Hernekamp JF. Enzymatic debridement for the treatment of severely burned upper extremities - early single center experiences. BMC Dermatology. 2016;**16**(1):8. DOI: 10.1186/s12895-016-0045-2

[29] De Freitas LR, Udoma-Udofa OC, Reginato PH, Mitsui HC, Provinciatto H, Torres FC. Bromelain-based enzymatic debridement versus standard of Care in Deep Burn Injuries: A systematic review and meta-analysis. Journal of Burn Care & Research. 2025;**46**(1):123-131. DOI: 10.1093/jbcr/irae172

[30] Hirche C, Kreken Almeland S, Dheansa B, Fuchs P, Governa M, Hoeksema H, et al. Eschar removal by bromelain based enzymatic debridement (Nexobrid®) in burns: European consensus guidelines update. Burns. 2020;**46**(4):782-796. DOI: 10.1016/j.burns.2020.03.002

[31] Sharaf A, Muthayya P. Microbial profile of burn wounds managed with enzymatic debridement using bromelain-based agent, NexoBrid®. Burns. 2022;**48**(7):1618-1625. DOI: 10.1016/j.burns.2021.12.004

[32] Mattern MM, Fuchs PC, Schiefer JL. Role, development, and value of enzymatic debridement as integral component in initial treatment of burn injuries exemplified by NexoBrid®. European Burn Journal. 2022;**3**(2):340-354. DOI: 10.3390/ebj3020029

[33] Tillett WS, Garner RL. The fibrinolytic activity of hemolytic streptococci. The Journal of Experimental Medicine. 1933;**58**(4):485-502. DOI: 10.1084/jem.58.4.485

[34] Tillett WS, Sherry S. The effect in patients of streptococcal fibrinolysin (streptokinase) and streptococcal desoxyribonuclease on fibrinous, purulent, and sanguinous pleural exudations. The Journal of Clinical Investigation. 1949;**28**(1):173-190. DOI: 10.1172/JCI102046

[35] Bond JS. Proteases: History, discovery, and roles in health and disease. The Journal of Biological Chemistry. 2019;**294**(5):1643-1651. DOI: 10.1074/jbc.TM118.004156

[36] Hummel RP, MacMillan BG, Maley M, Altemeier WA. Comparison of complete barrier isolation and unidirectional air flow isolation in the treatment of burn wounds. Annals of Surgery. 1972;**176**(6):742-747. DOI: 10.1097/00000658-197212000-00012

[37] Heinicke RM, Gortner WA. Stem bromelain—A new protease preparation from pineapple plants. Economic Botany. 1957;**11**:225-234. DOI: 10.1007/BF02860437

[38] Burke JF, Golden T. A clinical evaluation of enzymatic debridement with papain-urea-chlorophyllin ointment. American Journal of Surgery. 1958;**95**(5):828-842. DOI: 10.1016/0002-9610(58)90635-4

[39] Levine N, Seifter E, Connerton C, Levenson SM. Debridement of

experimental skin burns of pigs with bromelain, a pineapple-stem enzyme. Plastic and Reconstructive Surgery. 1973;**52**(4):413-424

[40] Levenson SM, Kan D, Gruber C, et al. Chemical debridement of burns. Annals of Surgery. 1974;**180**(4):670-704

[41] Houck JC, Chang CM, Klein G. Isolation of an effective debriding agent from the stems of pineapple plants. International Journal of Tissue Reactions. 1983;**5**(2):125-134

[42] Klein MB, Lezotte DL, Fauerbach JA, Herndon DN, Kowalske KJ, Carrougher GJ, et al. The National Institute on Disability and Rehabilitation Research burn model system database: A tool for the multicenter study of the outcome of burn injury. Journal of Burn Care & Research. 2007;**28**(1):84-96. DOI: 10.1097/BCR.0b013E31802C888E

[43] Shoham Y, Gasteratos K, Singer AJ, Krieger Y, Silberstein E, Goverman J. Bromelain-based enzymatic burn debridement: A systematic review of clinical studies on patient safety, efficacy and long-term outcomes. International Wound Journal. 2023;**20**(10):4364-4383. DOI: 10.1111/iwj.14308

[44] Rosenberg L, Krieger Y, Bogdanov-Berezovski A, Silberstein E, Shoham Y, Singer AJ. A novel rapid and selective enzymatic debridement agent for burn wound management: A multi-center RCT. Burns. 2014;**40**(3):466-474. DOI: 10.1016/j.burns.2013.08.013

[45] Snyder R, Hoffmeister T, Ead JK, Nass A, Klinger E, David-Zarbiv K, et al. Bromelain-based enzymatic debridement: Mechanism of action in the wound environment. A literature review. Wounds. 2024;**36**(12):429-436. DOI: 10.25270/wnds/24100

[46] Pertea M, Poroch V, Ciobanu P, Filip A, Velenciuc N, Lunca S, et al. Efficiency of bromelain-enriched enzyme mixture (NexoBrid™) in the treatment of burn wounds. Applied Sciences. 2021;**11**:8134. DOI: 10.3390/app11178134

[47] Aguirrezabala JA, Aguilera-Sáez J, Illa-Boixaderas M, Serracanta J, Monte-Soldado A, Rivas-Nicolls D, et al. Response of a single European burn center to Centelles mass casualty burn disaster: Enzymatic debridement utility. International Journal of Burns and Trauma. 2022;**12**(6):224-231

[48] Fitzhugh DJ, Shan S, Dewhirst MW, et al. Bromelain treatment decreases neutrophil migration to sites of inflammation. Clinical Immunology. 2008;**128**:66-74

[49] Taussig SJ, Batkin S. Bromelain, the enzyme complex of pineapple (Ananas comosus) and its clinical application. An update. Journal of Ethnopharmacology. 1988;**22**:191-203

[50] Batkin S, Taussig SJ, Szekerezes J. Antimetastatic effect of bromelain with or without its proteolytic and anticoagulant activity. Journal of Cancer Research and Clinical Oncology. 1988;**114**:507-508

[51] Hikisz P, Bernasinska-Slomczewska J. Beneficial properties of bromelain. Nutrients. 2021;**13**(12):4313. DOI: 10.3390/nu13124313

[52] Galeiras R, Mourelo M, Pértega S, López ME, Esmorís I. Procedural sedation and analgesia during enzymatic debridement of burn patients. Annals of Burns and Fire Disasters. 2018;**31**(3):223-227

[53] Hirche C, Citterio A, Hoeksema H, Koller J, Lehner M, Martinez JR, et al.

Eschar removal by bromelain based enzymatic debridement (Nexobrid®) in burns: An European consensus. Burns. 2017;**43**(8):1640-1653. DOI: 10.1016/j.burns.2017.07.025

[54] Shoham Y, Rosenberg L, Hickerson W, Goverman J, Iyer N, Barrera-Oro J, et al. Early enzymatic burn debridement: Results of the detect multicenter randomized controlled trial. Journal of Burn Care & Research. 2024;**45**(2):297-307. DOI: 10.1093/jbcr/irad142. Erratum in: J Burn Care Res. 2024 Jan 5;45(1):258. DOI: 10.1093/jbcr/irad155

[55] Harats M, Haik J, Cleary M, Vashurin I, Aviv U, Kornhaber R. A retrospective review of an off-label brome-lain-based selective enzymatic debridement (Nexobrid®) in the treatment of deep, partial, and full thickness burns and hard to heal wounds. The Israel Medical Association Journal: IMAJ. 2020;**22**:83-88

[56] Locci C, Chicconi E, Antonucci R. Current uses of bromelain in children: A narrative review. Children (Basel). 2024;**11**(3):377. DOI: 10.3390/children11030377

[57] Zuccaro J, Lee D, Kelly C, Chakera H, Turner E, Gus E, et al. A single institution's surgical care model for pediatric burns with ≤10% body surface area involvement. Journal of Burn Care & Research. 2025;**46**(1):22-27. DOI: 10.1093/jbcr/irae185

[58] European Medicines Agency. NexoBrid; 2024. [Online]. Available from: https://www.ema.europa.eu/en/medicines/human/EPAR/nexobrid [Accessed: February 5, 2024]

[59] Ferancikova N, Bukovcan P, Sarkozyova N, Dragunova J, Cucorova V, Koller J. Bromelain-based enzymatic debridement as a treatment of choice in high-risk patient with deep facial burns, a case report. International Journal of Surgery Case Reports. 2020;**71**:6-10. DOI: 10.1016/j.ijscr.2020.04.052

[60] Dadras M, Wagner JM, Wallner C, Sogorski A, Sacher M, Harati K, et al. Enzymatic debridement of hands with deep burns: A single center experience in the treatment of 52 hands. Journal of Plastic Surgery and Hand Surgery. 2020;**54**(4):220-224. DOI: 10.1080/2000656X.2020.1755298

[61] Corrales-Benítez C, González-Peinado D, González-Miranda Á, Martínez-Méndez JR. Evaluation of burned hand function after enzymatic debridement. Journal of Plastic, Reconstructive & Aesthetic Surgery. 2022;**75**(3):1048-1056. DOI: 10.1016/j.bjps.2021.09.074

[62] Lin Wu ZQ, Bulla A, Aguirrezabala Del Río JA, Rivas Nicolls DA, Aguilera Sáez J, Serracanta Domènech J, et al. Enzymatic debridement (Nexobrid) on burned hands: Retrospective review from a burn referral center in Spain. Plastic and Reconstructive Surgery. Global Open. 2024;**12**(6):e5886. DOI: 10.1097/GOX.0000000000005886

[63] Rivas-Nicolls D, Aguilera-Sáez J, Gallardo-Calero I, Serracanta J, Gomez P, Palao R, et al. Does enzymatic debridement allow us to perform conservative treatment on clinically deep hand burns? A retrospective review. Annals of Burns and Fire Disasters. 2020;**33**(3):239-244

[64] Malsagova AT, El-Habbassi A, Billner M, Berns M, Pueski T, Bodenschatz KJ, et al. Long-term functional outcomes following enzymatic debridement of deep hand burns using Nexobrid®: A retrospective analysis. Journal of Clinical Medicine.

2024;**13**(16):4729. DOI: 10.3390/jcm13164729

[65] Krieger Y, Rubin G, Schulz A, Rosenberg N, Levi A, Singer AJ, et al. Bromelain-based enzymatic debridement and minimal invasive modality (mim) care of deeply burned hands. Annals of Burns and Fire Disasters. 2017;**30**(3):198-204

[66] Mataro I, Lanza A, Di Franco S, Di Franco L, Sangiuolo M, Notaro M, et al. Releasing burn-induced compartment syndrome by enzymatic escharotomy-debridement: A case study. Journal of Burn Care & Research. 2020;**41**(5):1097-1103. DOI: 10.1093/jbcr/iraa055

[67] Fischer S, Haug V, Diehm Y, Rhodius P, Cordts T, Schmidt VJ, et al. Feasibility and safety of enzymatic debridement for the prevention of operative escharotomy in circumferential deep burns of the distal upper extremity. Surgery. 2019;**165**(6):1100-1105. DOI: 10.1016/j.surg.2018.11.019

[68] Grünherz L, Michienzi R, Schaller C, Rittirsch D, Uyulmaz S, Kim BS, et al. Enzymatic debridement for circumferential deep burns: The role of surgical escharotomy. Burns. 2023;**49**(2):304-309. DOI: 10.1016/j.burns.2022.12.003

[69] Jeschke MG, van Baar ME, Choudhry MA, Chung KK, Gibran NS, Logsetty S. Burn injury. Nature Reviews Disease Primers. 2020;**6**(1):11. DOI: 10.1038/s41572-020-0145-5

[70] Yakupu A, Zhang J, Dong W, Song F, Dong J, Lu S. The epidemiological characteristic and trends of burns globally. BMC Public Health. 2022;**22**(1):1596. DOI: 10.1186/s12889-022-13887-2

[71] Agrawal P, Nikhade P, Patel A, Mankar N, Sedani S. Bromelain: A potent phytomedicine. Cureus. 2022;**14**(8):e27876. DOI: 10.7759/cureus.27876

[72] Leelakanok N, Petchsomrit A, Janurai T, Saechan C, Sunsandee N. Efficacy and safety of bromelain: A systematic review and meta-analysis. Nutrition and Health. 2023;**29**(3):479-503. DOI: 10.1177/02601060231173732

[73] Jančič U, Gorgieva S. Bromelain and nisin: The natural antimicrobials with high potential in biomedicine. Pharmaceutics. 2021;**14**(1):76. DOI: 10.3390/pharmaceutics14010076

[74] Bahar R, Chegeni MJ, Tahvildari A, Sani M, Khakpour Y, Hashemabady M, et al. Bromelain decreases oxidative stress and neuroinflammation and improves motor function in adult male rats with cerebellar Ataxia induced by 3-acetylpyridine. Neuropeptides. 2024;**107**:102455. DOI: 10.1016/j.npep.2024.102455

[75] Martinez-Mendez J-R et al. Consensus guideline about the use of the enzimatic debridement in burn injuries with NexoBrid®. Cir Plást. Iberolatinoam. 2017;**43**(2):193-202. ISSN 1989-2055

[76] Serracanta J, Baena J, Martinez-Mendez JR, Sanchez-Sanchez M, Lopez-Suso E, Galeiras R, et al. Bromelain-based enzymatic burn debridement: Spanish multidisciplinary consensus. European Journal of Plastic Surgery. 2023;**46**(2):271-279. DOI: 10.1007/s00238-022-01999-2

[77] Gonzalez L, Gonzalez R, Callejas I, Roig G, Seoane N, Minguez S, et al. Consensus on the application and care of bromelain-based enzymatic debridement on burns. Annals of Burns and Fire Disasters. 2024;**37**(3):208-216

[78] Ranno R, Vestita M, Maggio G, Verrienti P, Melandri D, Orlandi C, et al. Italian recommendations on enzymatic debridement in burn surgery. Burns. 2021;**47**(2):408-416. DOI: 10.1016/j.burns.2020.07.006

[79] Korzeniowski T, Strużyna J, Chrapusta AM, Krajewski A, Kucharzewski M, Piorun K, et al. A questionnaire-based study to obtain a consensus from 5 Polish burns centers on eschar removal by bromelain-based enzymatic debridement (Nexobrid®) in burns following the 2020 updated European consensus guidelines. Medical Science Monitor. 2022;**28**:e935632. DOI: 10.12659/MSM.935632

[80] Marinescu SA. A new bromelain-enriched proteolytic enzymes concentrate treatment in patients with extensive burns: Romanian consensus. Farmácia. 2021;**69**(4):792-798

[81] Zamani KA. Are burn patients satisfied with anesthesia in enzymatic debridement? Burns. 2022;**48**(8):2002-2003. DOI: 10.1016/j.burns.2022.09.008

[82] Schiefer JL, Lipensky A, Fuchs PC, Heitzmann W, Schulz A. Patients' satisfaction with anesthesia in enzymatic debridement from a surgical perspective. Burns. 2020;**46**(5):1073-1082. DOI: 10.1016/j.burns.2019.11.003

[83] Capitelli-McMahon H, McCrossan S, Kershaw J, Muthayya P, Anwar MU, Carter A, et al. The use of NexoBrid™ enzymatic debridement and coagulation abnormalities. Burns. 2024;**50**(1):123-131. DOI: 10.1016/j.burns.2023.06.012

Chapter 5

Low-Intensity Extracorporeal Shock Wave Therapy in the Management of Wound Healing

Jens J. Rassweiler, Juvido Agatep, Clarice Condeno and Wolfgang Schaden

Abstract

Wound healing is an intricate biological process characterized by phases of inflammation, tissue proliferation, and remodeling, all aimed at restoring the integrity of damaged tissues. Chronic wounds and ulcers are particularly troublesome, as they often heal incompletely and have a high likelihood of recurrence, presenting substantial difficulties for standard treatment approaches. Recently, extracorporeal shock wave therapy (ESWT) has gained traction as a promising intervention for facilitating wound healing. In this review, we examine the current knowledge surrounding ESWT for wound management, drawing from personal experiences and an extensive review of existing literature. This therapy utilizes either focused or radial shock waves to stimulate the healing process through mechanisms such as angiogenesis, fibroblast proliferation, and enhanced collagen synthesis. Evidence gathered from systematic reviews indicates that ESWT leads to favorable outcomes in wound healing, including improved healing rates and significant reductions in wound size for chronic conditions like diabetic foot ulcers, pressure sores, and venous ulcers. Furthermore, ESWT has demonstrated a favorable safety profile, with only minor and transient side effects reported, such as mild pain, swelling, and redness at the treatment site. Consequently, ESWT offers a noninvasive and safe alternative for addressing various challenges associated with wound healing, ultimately enhancing the quality of life for patients suffering from chronic wounds and ulcers, including those with Fournier's gangrene, particularly in postoperative contexts.

Keywords: extracorporeal shock wave therapy, Fournier's gangrene, decubitus, wound healing, stem-cell proliferation, re-epithelialization

1. Introduction

Extracorporeal shock waves have been used since 1980 in medicine. Primarily, high-energy shock waves have been applied to disintegrate renal stones [1, 2] and lately to treat Peyronie's disease [3, 4] or pseudoarthrosis [5]. In the early 1980s of the last century, the concept of low-intensity extracorporeal shock wave therapy (Li-ESWT) was developed mainly in the field of orthopedics [6], stimulated by the success of extracorporeal shock wave lithotripsy (ESWL). First trials on the application of Li-ESWT for the management of wound healing started in the early years of this century [7]. Unlike the use of shock waves for stone fragmentation (ESWL), when treating soft tissue diseases, only low energy flux density is required. Thus, low-intensity extracorporeal shock wave therapy (Li-ESWT) has less than 0.35 mJ/ mm^2 per impulse [8].

Already in 1990, Haupt et al. [9] examined the effect of shock waves on wound healing in an *in vivo* porcine model using the Dornier XL1 experimental lithotripter and concluded that lower energy levels (14 vs. 18 kV generator voltage) resulted in an increased vascularization. More than 10 years later, in 2007, Schaden et al. [7] initiated the first clinical trial on Li-ESWT on wound healing.

In this chapter, we want to present an overview of the actual use of Li-ESWT in the management of wound healing and, based on recent personal experiences, discuss further options and possible applications of this noninvasive technology [10].

2. Problems of wound healing

Wound healing is a complex process involving inflammation, proliferation, and tissue remodeling, which ultimately restores the integrity of damaged tissue [11]. While most wounds close within weeks, disruption of the healing process can lead to chronic wounds or ulcers, characterized by incomplete or prolonged healing with a high risk of recurrence [12]. Various factors, including local causes like infection and tissue hypoxia, systemic diseases like diabetes mellitus, and certain medications, contribute to the development of chronic wounds such as diabetic ulcers, venous leg ulcers, or pressure ulcers [13].

Managing chronic wounds requires addressing the primary cause, such as controlling blood sugar levels in diabetics or vascular surgery for patients with venous or ischemic vascular disease [11]. Additional treatments involve the removal of necrotic or infected tissue, including wound cleansing and proper diet. Compression therapy is particularly relevant for venous leg ulcers, as it improves venous return [12, 13]. Despite these measures, many chronic wounds fail to heal or recur, prompting the search for new effective treatment options, such as hyperbaric oxygen therapy (HBO) [14].

3. Technical background of shock waves

Shock waves are mechanical, acoustic waves distinguished by their high-pressure amplitudes and abrupt pressure increases [15]. Unlike conventional ultrasound, which consists of periodic oscillations with limited bandwidth, shock waves can encompass a broad range of frequencies, typically from a few kilohertz (kHz) to over 10 megahertz (MHz). There are two primary types of shock waves, categorized based on the technology used for their generation (**Figure 1**).

Focused shock waves can be generated by means of electrohydraulic, piezoelectric, or electromagnetic shock wave generators [15]. They have to be distinguished from unfocused radial shock waves [16, 17].

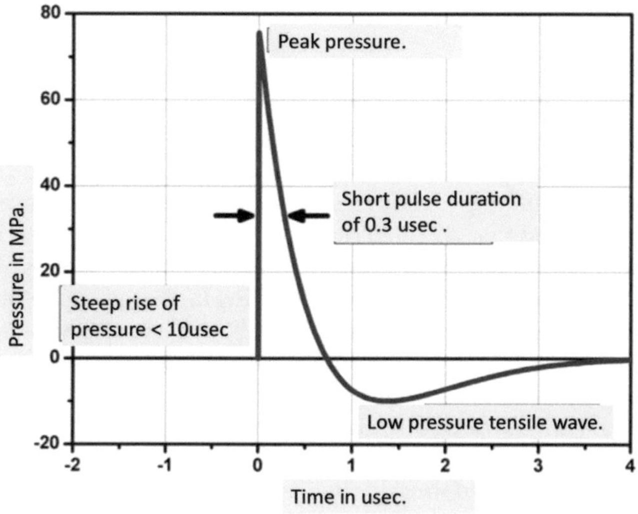

Figure 1.
Pressure curve of a shock wave with a short duration (<10 μs) consisting of a compressive phase (peak pressure 30–100 MPa) followed by a tensile phase.

i. Electrohydraulic shock wave generation: This method relies on a spark initiated by a high voltage applied between two electrode tips positioned at the focal point of a parabolic reflector. The spark causes rapid vaporization of the water between the tips, resulting in the creation of a spherical shock wave. This technique allows for the delivery of shock wave energy over a large coupling area due to the relatively large aperture of the shock wave source compared to the focal size. However, the majority of the shock wave energy is concentrated within a relatively small focal zone inside the body.

ii. Electromagnetic shock wave generation: This approach utilizes the principles of electromagnetic induction. Electromagnetic devices often employ a cylindrical coil to generate shock waves, which are then focused using a rotational paraboloid design.

iii. Piezoelectric shock wave sources use the curved arrangement of piezoelectric crystals to create a self-focusing system. This technology also allows the production of linear shock waves [16].

iv. Radial pressure waves are created by a ballistic pressure wave system, which is based on the linear impulse-momentum principle deduced from Newton's law [16]. These shock waves are characterized by a dominant, primarily positive pressure pulse, typically followed by smaller tensile wave components. The positive pressure pulse lasts approximately 0.3–0.5 microseconds (μs), while the total duration of the pulse is about three times longer, approximately 1–2 μs [17]. Typical peak pressures for radial pressure waves range from about 0.1–1 megapascal (MPa). Although radial pressure waves are unfocused and cannot reach deep tissues in the body, this characteristic is not problematic for applications related to wound management.

4. Mechanism of low-energy shock wave therapy

Based on early studies of Haupt et al. in 1992 [9], several animal studies have been performed to evaluate the potential of ESWT for the treatment of wounds. In mouse and rat burn wound models, ESWT was found to induce angiogenesis and to enhance the percentage of wound closure, the re-epithelialization rates, blood flow, and the number of rolling and sticking leukocytes, suggesting improved metabolism [18].

It was further reported that repeated sessions accelerate angiogenesis in burn wounds significantly more than a single application [19]. The angiogenic effects of ESWT were confirmed in a murine skin graft model, also showing increased expression of VEGF-A and other cytokines involved in angiogenesis [20]. ESWT can also activate key factors involved in connective tissue repair, such as fibroblasts that increase proliferation and expression of essential factors like TGF-beta-1 and collagen types I and III [21, 22].

Thus, its primary mechanism of action in the management of wounds is believed to be improving tissue circulation by stimulating the production of energy-rich nitric oxide (NO), leading to reduced muscle rigidity and improved biomechanical functioning, enhancing mobility and self-perception [18–22]. However, recent trials using ESWT for improvement of wound healing after Fournier's gangrene also indicate a stimulation of local stem cells [23, 24].

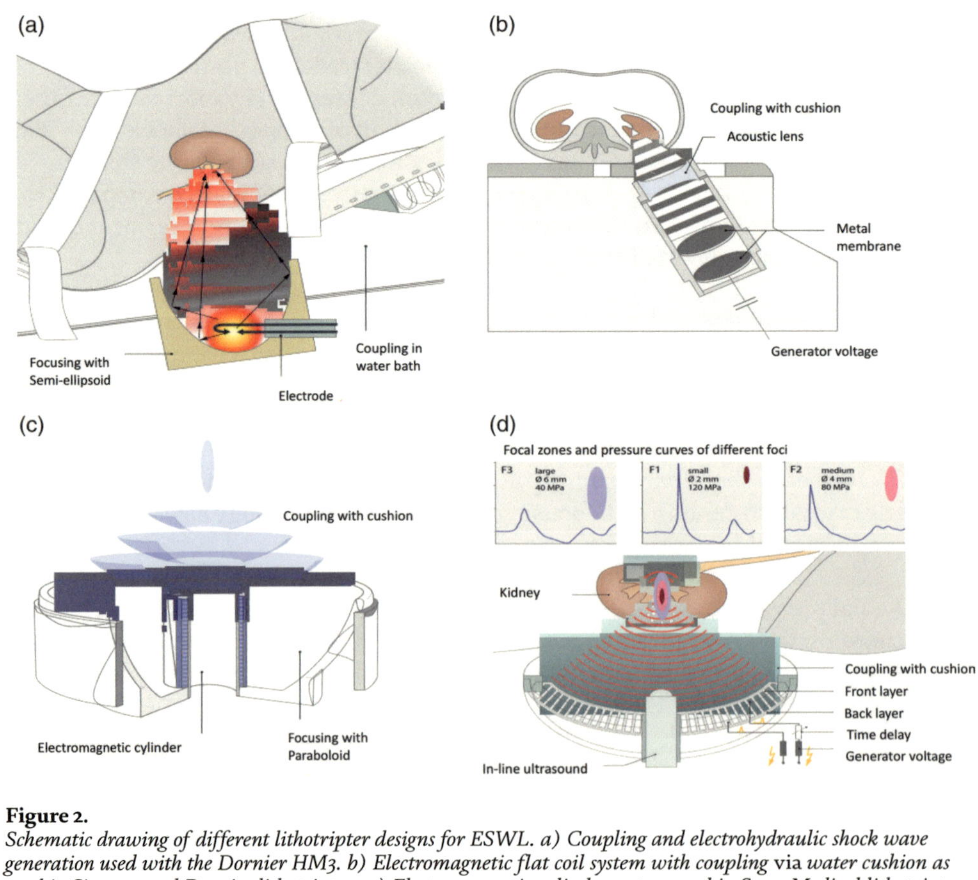

Figure 2.
Schematic drawing of different lithotripter designs for ESWL. a) Coupling and electrohydraulic shock wave generation used with the Dornier HM3. b) Electromagnetic flat coil system with coupling via *water cushion as used in Siemens and Dornier lithotripters. c) Electromagnetic cylinder system used in Storz Medical lithotripters. d) Piezoelectric shockwave generation using two layers of piezo-ceramic elements used in Wolf Piezolith 3000 with technical realization of three different focal zones.*

Whereas high-energy shock waves used for lithotripsy use mechanical forces created by the interface of urine-stone, resulting in fragmentation of the stone, the mechanism of low-intensity shock waves is believed to be based on an effect on the cellular base, called *mechano-transduction* [25]. The process of mechano-transduction refers to a cellular mechanism by which load-bearing cells sense physical forces, transduce the forces into biochemical signals, and generate appropriate responses leading to alterations in cellular structure and function. Such signal transduction pathways being activated in response to mechanical forces include many unique components as well as elements shared by other signaling pathways [25]. In this scenario, shock waves are an ideal tool to induce the process of mechano-transduction in any part of the body in a noninvasive way (**Figure 2**).

Mechano-transduction is a biological mechanism through which cells convert mechanical forces into biochemical signals. Various signal transduction pathways can be activated in response to these mechanical forces, featuring numerous unique components alongside elements shared with other signaling pathways.

In this context, shock waves serve as an effective tool for inducing mechano-transduction processes throughout the body in a noninvasive manner. To facilitate this, manufacturers have developed handheld devices specifically designed for delivering shock waves to targeted areas of the body.

5. Treatment parameters of Li-ESWT

Table 1 summarizes the treatment data applied in the reviews reported on the use of extracorporeal shock wave therapy in the treatment of the indications of acute and chronic wounds, including burns, postburn scars, venous ulcers, pressure ulcers, decubitus ulcers, diabetic foot ulcers, and gangrene, primarily affecting the limbs and extremities. Most treatments with ESWT involved multiple treatment sessions, and there was a range of values applied for the technical parameters of the devices [23, 24, 26–30, 32].

In essence, depending on the size of the wound, 2000–3000 shock waves per session are applied with a handheld device (**Figure 2**) at a frequency of 4–5 Hz using an

Indication	Energy flux density [mJ/mm²]	Frequency [Hz]	Impulses [*pulses/cm²*]	Sessions
Burns/burn scars [26]	0.05–0.23	4	100	1-6
Burn scars [27]	0.03–0.25	NR	100–600	1–10
Chronic wounds (CWLE) [28]	0.03–0.25	NR	100–600	1–10
Diabetic foot ulcer [29–31]	0.03–0.23	4–5	100–500	3–20
Mixed ulcers (PU/VU/DFU) [32, 33]	0.03–0.27	4–5	25–500	1–10
Fournier's gangrene [23, 24]	0.25	3–4	100–200	5–18
Decubitus with fistula*	0.25–0.34	4	200–500	30
Overall range for all indications	*0.03–0.34*	*4–5*	*25–600*	*1–30*

*Abbreviations: CWLE: Chronic wounds of the lower extremity; DFU: Diabetic foot ulcer; NR: Not reported; PBS: Postburn scars; PU: Pressure ulcers; VU: Venous ulcer. *Present study.*

Table 1.
Range of parameter data for low-intensity extracorporeal shock wave therapy of wounds identified in the literature (modified from Rassweiler et al. [10]).

energy flux density of 0.03–0.34 mJ/mm^2. This corresponds to 25–600 impulses per cm^2 of the wound. At this energy level, there is no need for anesthesia or analgesia.

6. Parameters to evaluate the use of Li-ESWT for wound healing

There are multiple reviews that reported on extracorporeal shock wave therapy (ESWT) for the cellular treatment of various acute and chronic wounds. This includes conditions such as burns, postburn scars, venous ulcers, pressure ulcers, decubitus ulcers, diabetic foot ulcers, and gangrene, primarily affecting the limbs and extremities.

Most ESWT treatments involve multiple sessions, with a range of applied values. Specifically, depending on the size of the wound, 2000–3000 shock waves are delivered per session using a handheld device (**Figure 3**). The treatment is administered at a frequency of 4–5 Hz, employing specific technical parameters outlined in **Table 1**. The energy flux density applied ranges from 0.03 to 0.34 mJ/mm^2, which corresponds to delivering 25–600 impulses per cm^2 of the wound area. Importantly, treatments at this energy level do not necessitate anesthesia or analgesia for patients [23, 24, 26–30, 32].

Outcomes for the treatment of burn scars included assessment of specific performance, such as pain, pruritus, scar appearance score (VSS), scar thickness, scar elasticity, and trans-epidermal water loss [23, 24, 26–30, 32].

Table 2 summarizes the performance data reported across all 11 systematic reviews, indicating a consistent positive clinical effect of Li-ESWT when combined with standard wound care [26–32, 35–37].

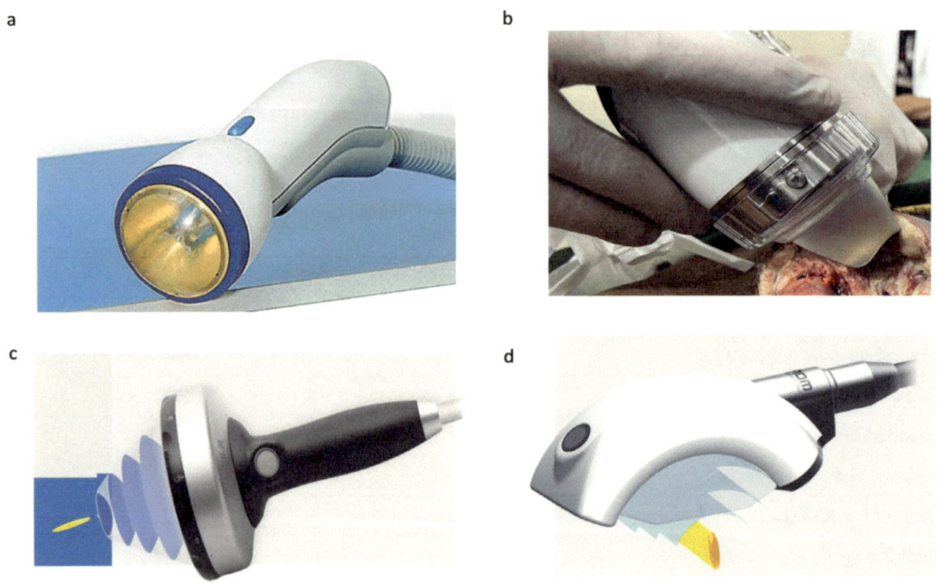

Figure 3.
Different handheld devices for Li-ESWT. a) Electrohydraulic device Urogold 100 (MTS, Konstanz, Germany). b) Electromagnetic device Duolith SD (Storz Medical, Taegerwilen, Switzerland). c) Piezoelectric device Piezowave 2 (Elvation, Knittlingen, Germany) handpiece for focal ESWT. d) Piezoelectric device Piezowave 2 (Elvation, Knittlingen, Germany) handpiece for linear ESWT.

DOI: http://dx.doi.org/10.5772/intechopen.1012959

Reference	Aim	Study details	Intervention(s)	Outcomes	Authors' conclusions
a) Burns					
Aguilera-Sáez J et al. [26]	To review the literature for published evidence on the use of ESWT for the treatment of acute burn patients	14 studies (5 RCTs) • Acute burns • Post-burn scars • Post-burn heterotopic ossification	ESWT (Extracorporeal shock wave therapy) + Standard Care (14 studies) *ESWT protocols:* *0.05–0.23 mJ/mm², 4 Hz, 1–6 sessions; 100 SW/cm²*	• VSS • TTE • Scar thickness • Pain • Pruritus	ESWT seems to be a promising tool in this field, and therefore, more high-quality trials should be conducted.
Yang Y et al. [27]	To evaluate the efficacy of ESWT and rehabilitation therapy on postburn scars compared to rehabilitation therapy alone	9 studies (n = 422) • Post-burn scars	ESWT + Standard Care (9 studies) *ESWT protocols:* *0.03–0.25 mJ/mm², 4 Hz, 1–10 sessions;100–500 SW/cm²*	• Pain • Thickness • Pruritus • Adverse events	Mild-to-moderate evidence for the use of ESWT as an adjuvant therapy to the standard wound care program.
b) Diabetic foot ulcers					
Hitchman LH, et al. [29]	To assess available evidence on the efficacy of ESWT for the healing of diabetic foot ulcers	5 studies (n = 255) • Diabetic foot ulcers	ESWT + Standard Care (5 studies) HBO + Standard Care (2 studies) *ESWT protocols:* *0.03–0.2 mJ/mm², 4–5 Hz, 3–16 sessions; 100–500 SW/cm²*	• Healing/RE (%, time) • QoL • Adverse events (incl. infection)	ESWT has the potential to improve healing in diabetic foot ulcers, although there is insufficient evidence to justify its use in clinical routine.
Huang Q, et al. [30]	To assess the efficacy and safety of ESWT on the healing of diabetic foot ulcers	8 studies (n = 339) • Diabetic foot ulcers	ESWT + Standard Care (8 studies) HBO + Standard Care (2 studies) *ESWT protocols:* *0.03–0.23 mJ/mm², 4 Hz, 3–8 sessions;100–500 SW/cm²,*	• Healing/RE (%, time) • SA/closure • Adverse events	ESWT can effectively improve the complete cure rate, shorten the healing period, and significantly enhance treatment efficacy.

Reference	Aim	Study details	Intervention(s)	Outcomes	Authors' conclusions
Hitchman, L., et al. [31]	To appraise the evidence on the role of ESWT in diabetic foot ulcer healing and the impact of different ESWT doses	6 studies (n = 471) • Diabetic foot ulcers	ESWT + Standard Care (6 studies) Standard Care ± sham (6 studies) *ESWT protocols:* *0.03–0.23 mJ/mm², 4 Hz, 3–20 sessions; 100–500 SW/cm²*	• Healing/RE (%, time) • SA/closure • QoL • Adverse events	Patients treated with ESWT were more likely to heal at 20 weeks post-ESWT compared to standard ulcer care alone.
c) Different types of wounds					
Dymarek R, et al. [34]	To evaluate available evidence of ESWT in human wounds	13 studies (n = 919) • Wounds • Post-surgical wounds • Diabetic foot ulcers • Pressure ulcers	ESWT + Standard Care (13 studies) HBO + Standard Care (2 studies) *ESWT protocols:* *0.03–0.23 mJ/mm², 4–5 Hz, 1–6 sessions, 25–500 SW/cm²*	• Healing/RE • (%, time) • Severity • SA/closure • Adverse events	In the controlled clinical studies, statistically significant differences in rates of wound closure were observed compared to a variety of standard topical treatment modalities, sham ESWT treatment, and HBO.
Butterworth, PA, et al. [35]	To investigate the effectiveness of ESWT for the treatment of lower limb ulceration	5 studies (n = 249) • Ulcers of lower limb, • Venous ulcers • Diabetic foot ulcers	ESWT + Standard Care (n = 149, 5 studies) HBO + Standard Care (n = 75, 2 studies) *ESWT protocols:* *0.03–0.27 mJ/mm², 4 Hz, 1–10 sessions, 100 SW/cm²*	• Healing/RE • (%, time) • Severity • SA/closure • Adverse events	Only limited evidence was identified. Further research is needed to support the use of extracorporeal shock wave therapy in the treatment of lower limb ulceration.
Omar MT, et al. [28]	Review the efficacy of ESWT on the healing of chronic wounds on the lower extremity	11 studies (n = 925): • Chronic wounds of lower extremity	ESWT + Standard Care (11 studies) HBO + Standard Care (2 studies) *ESWT protocols:* *0.03–0.25 mJ/mm², 4 Hz, 1–10 sessions, 100–600 SW/cm²*	• Healing/RE (%, time) • SA/closure • Adverse events	Mild-to-moderate evidence to support the use of ESWT as an adjuvant therapy with a standardized wound care program.

Reference	Aim	Study details	Intervention(s)	Outcomes	Authors' conclusions
Dolibog P et al. [36]	Current state of knowledge on the use of shockwave therapy in the treatment of soft tissue wounds	14 studies • Burns • Diabetic foot ulcers • Venous ulcers • Pressure ulcers • Gangrene	ESWT + Standard Care (14 studies) HBO (1 study) *ESWT protocols:* *0.03–0.25 mJ/mm^2, 4–5 Hz, 1–30 sessions,100–2000 SW/cm^2*	• Healing/RE (%) • Severity • SA/closure • Adverse events	Evidence suggests a beneficial effect of ESWT to treat diabetic foot ulcers, venous leg ulcers, pressure ulcers, and burns.
Zhang, L., et al. [32]	Effectiveness of ESWT compared to the standard care treatment for the healing of chronic wounds	7 studies (n = 301) • Chronic Wounds • Diabetic foot ulcers • Decubitus ulcers	ESWT + Standard Care (7 studies) Standard Care + HBO (2 studies) *ESWT protocols:* *0.03–0.23 mJ/mm^2, 4–5 Hz, 3–8 sessions, 100–500 SW/cm^2*	• Healing/RE (%, time) • SA/closure • Adverse events (incl. Infection, pain)	ESWT as an adjunct to wound treatment improves the healing process of chronic wounds more than the standard care treatment alone.
Zhang, L., et al. [37]	To compare the effects of ESWT and conventional wound therapy for acute and chronic soft tissue wounds	10 studies (n = 473) • Wounds (acute/chronic) • Burns • Diabetic foot ulcers	ESWT + Standard Care (10 studies) Standard Care + HBO (2 studies) *ESWT protocols:* *0.03–0.23 mJ/mm^2, 4–5 Hz, 1–8 sessions, 25–500 pulses/cm^2*	• Healing/RE (%, time) • SA/closure • Adverse events (incl. infection)	ESWT showed better therapeutic effects on acute and chronic soft tissue wounds compared to conventional wound therapy.

Abbreviations: ESWT = Extracorporeal shock wave therapy; HBO = Hyperbaric oxygen therapy; RE = Re-epithelialization; SA = Surface area. SW = pulses of shocks.

Table 2.
Outcome data of relevant systematic reviews and meta-analyses for the use of Li-ESWT for wound healing differentiated according to the type of lesion (modified from Rassweiler et al. [10]).

The outcomes evaluated included wound healing progression, the proportion of completely healed wounds, healing time, healing rate, and reduction in wound area/percentage of healed wound area, as well as the incidence of unresponsive wounds, recurring wounds, and infection rates.

7. Detailed effects of Li-ESWT on wound healing

Based on these criteria, Li-ESWT has demonstrated positive clinical performance for various types of wounds, including diabetic foot ulcers (**Figure 4**), pressure ulcers, venous ulcers, decubitus ulcers, chronic wounds, acute burn wounds, postburn scars, and postburn heterotopic ossification [26–32, 35–37]. A summary of key clinical performance outcomes identified from the systematic reviews for the treatment of postburn scars is presented in **Table 2**.

The systematic reviews noted one alternative treatment option, hyperbaric oxygen therapy (HBO), which has been specifically used for the treatment of diabetic foot ulcers [29, 30, 32]. In this group, ESWT proved to be superior (**Table 3**).

Moreover, recent studies using ESWT in postoperative wound management of Fournier's gangrene by Rassweiler et al. [23, 24] showed complete restoration of the skin defect with adequate local skin tissue regeneration (i.e., penile vs. scrotal vs. gluteal) with no side effects for the patients (**Figures 2** and **3**).

Additionally, we had a very interesting case treating a decubitus with two fistulas in the gluteal area in a paraplegic patient, who was already a candidate for a large plastic surgery. Within 3 months, we were able to close all fistulas and to reduce the size of the decubitus remarkably, inducing an ongoing process of tissue regeneration in the subcutis around the shrinking decubitus (**Figure 4**).

a

b

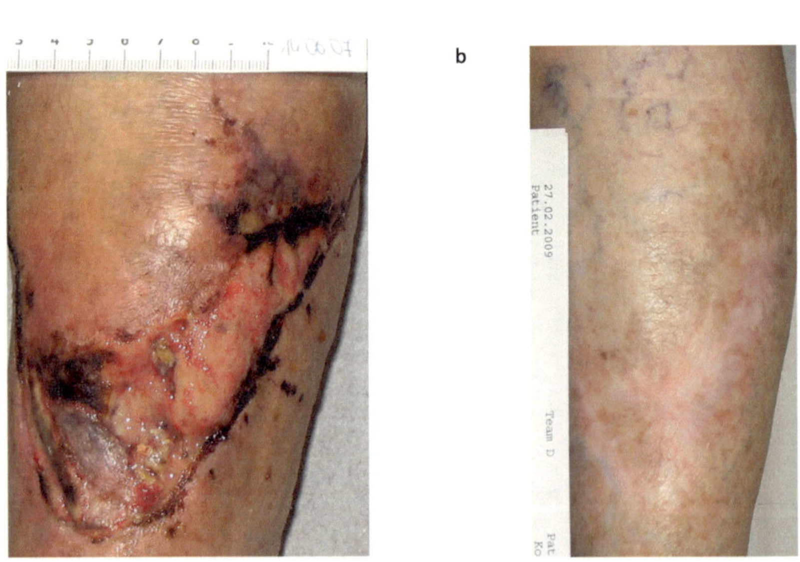

Figure 4.
An 82-year-old female with diabetic foot syndrome. Complete healing after three treatments with low-intensity extracorporeal shock wave therapy (Li-ESWT) using an electrohydraulic focal shock wave generator (2300 impulses at 4 Hz). a) Initial finding with a large ulcer resistant to classical wound dressing. b) Complete healing of the wound with minimal scar formation after 3 months.

Parameter	Studies	Li-ESWT	HBO	ESWT vs. HBO	Reference
Healed ulcers (complete)	4 (n = 156)	• RR = 1.83; 95% CI, 1.14–2.94; p = 0.012 (vs HBO)		Improvement, 1.8-fold	Huang et al. [30]
Healed ulcers (complete)	2 (ESWT = 80, SWC = 76)	• 30.6%-54.5%	• 22.2%-25.0%	Improvement, 2.4-fold	Hitchman et al. [29]
		• OR = 2.45 [95% Cl: 1.03–6.87], p = 0.03			
Unresponsive ulcers	4 (n = 156)	• RR = 0.25; 95% CI, 0.13–0.48; p < 0.001		Improvement, 4-fold	Huang et al. [30]
Healing rate of ulcers	5 (ESWT = 80, SWC = 76)	• 50–88.9%	• 0%-72.2%	Improvement 2.7-fold	Zhang et al. [32]
		• OR = 2.77 [95% Cl: 1.34–4.71], p = 0.006			
		• OR = 2.77 [95% Cl: 1.34–4.71], p = 0.006			

SWC = Standard wound care; Li-ESWT = low-intensity extracorporeal shock wave therapy.

Table 3.
Data on performance outcomes for diabetic foot ulcers treated with Li-ESWT compared to hyperbaric oxygen therapy (HBO) from systematic reviews (modified from Rassweiler et al. [10]).

8. Side effects of Li-ESWT

In reviews of Li-ESWT, reports of infection indicated that the incidence in the ESWT group was similar to or lower than that in the standard care comparator group [26–32, 35, 36]. The most frequently reported safety events associated with Li-ESWT were transient and mild, including:

- Reddish discoloration of the skin
- Bruising
- Swelling
- Small hematomas
- Petechiae
- Edema at the treatment site
- Mild pain or discomfort during treatment

Systematic review	Safety event
Hitchman [31]	Safety events in 4 of 6 included studies of diabetic foot ulcers • Infection: ESWT: 28–36.8% vs. Control: 25.3–35.8% • Amputation: ESWT: 2.3% vs. Control: 3.0%
Yang [27]	Safety events in 3 of 9 included studies • Transitory reddening and edema of the skin • Mild-to-moderate pain • No serious adverse events
Aguilera-Sáez [26]	No reported safety events in 9 included studies
Huang [30]	Safety events in 5 of 8 included studies • Transitory reddening of the skin • Slight pain • Small hematomas
Hitchman [29]	No reported safety events in 7 included studies
Zhang [37]	Safety events in 6 of 12 included studies • Transitory reddening of the skin • Slight pain • Small hematomas
Doliborg [36]	Safety events in 9 of 11 included studies during treatment • Infection: ESWT: 28–36.8%, vs. Control: 25.3–35.8%) • Increase in pressure ulcer size during treatment: n = 3 • Mild pain during application (ulcers) • Infection: ESWT: 9%, vs. Control: 14% • Microtrauma, swelling, bruising, petechiae, as well as pain (before, during, and after treatment)

Systematic review	Safety event
Zhang [32]	• No serious adverse events in 7 included studies
Omar [28]	Safety events in 10 of 11 included studies • Pain • Itching • Skin irritation/pigmentation • Local infection (n = 1 in ESWT and Control groups; Moretti et al.) • (HBO: middle ear barotraumas and sinus pain)
Butterworth [35]	Safety events in 3 of 5 included studies • No serious adverse events in 5 included studies
Dymarek [34]	Safety events in 3 of 7 included studies • Local signs of infection (n = 1) • Wound infection rates: • 9% with ESWT vs. 14% with standard wound care • Enlarged ulcers with ischemic edges (n = 3)

Table 4.
Identified safety events reported in systematic reviews on the use of Li-ESWT in wound management (modified from Rassweiler et al. [10]).

The serious adverse events reported included infection and amputation. However, such complications were not caused by ESWT. Infection rates were noted to occur in up to 36.8% of patients treated for ulcers and up to 9% for those treated for burns with ESWT (**Table 4**).

While localized safety events specifically for ESWT treatment were not comprehensively reported, it is worth noting that hyperbaric oxygen therapy (HBO) was associated with several adverse effects, such as middle ear barotraumas and sinus pain [29, 30, 32].

Overall, ESWT was well-tolerated and did not prove to have a causal association with any serious adverse events reported in the literature.

9. Recommendation of Li-ESWT in guidelines

The DIGEST guideline [8] supports the use of extracorporeal shock wave therapy (ESWT), primarily advocating its application for the treatment of burn wounds and scars (**Table 5**). Also, ISMST guidelines are dealing with wound healing: https://shockwavetherapy.org/wp-content/uploads/2024/01/ISMST-Guidelines-for-ESWT-_-engl-20240103.pdf

10. Discussion

Recent studies have highlighted the positive effects of low-intensity extracorporeal shock wave therapy (Li-ESWT) in the treatment of chronic wounds, particularly in the context of pseudarthroses on the lower leg [5]. A pilot trial involving 208 patients with various wound healing disorders demonstrated that wounds treated with ESWT achieved complete epithelialization significantly faster than those in the placebo group [38].

Post-market experience and clinical evaluations of ESWT devices have shown only a few minor safety events, reinforcing the notion that ESWT is a very safe treatment

Reference	Scope/aim	Populations/indications	Relevance for clinical evaluation
ISMST, *DIGEST Guidelines for Extracorporeal Shock Wave Therapy*. 2019[1]	Guidance providing evidence-based background on clinical use of ESWT and treatment recommendations.	Any patient affected by burn injuries (including skin and internal injury from thermal, chemical, electrical, or toxic/ inhalation) in any patient. *Indications* • Wounds • Burn injuries • Burn scars	ESWT is recommended for use with: • Wounds, including burn injuries and burn scars, in conjunction with conservative treatment for 1st-2nd degree (class a) burns, or after initial surgical wound treatment for 2nd(class b)-4th degree burns. Significant improvements were reported for mesh-graft removal site healing and 2a° burns as well as burn scars, consistent with preclinical study reports. • Burn scars: Healing speed (rESWT) and perfusion (ESWT), pain (fESWT: 0.05-0.15 mJ/ mm2, 2000 impulses, three sessions, 4 Hz),)

[1]*https://shockwavetherapy.org/wp-content/uploads/2024/01/ISMST-Guidelines-for-ESWT-_-engl-20240103.pdf*

Table 5.
Overview of a relevant guideline identified in the literature (modified from Rassweiler et al. [10]).

option for patients [26–33, 35, 36, 39]. The systematic reviews available primarily noted hyperbaric oxygen therapy (HBO) as an alternative treatment option; however, it is associated with several adverse effects, such as middle ear barotrauma or sinus pain [29, 30, 32]. Overall, the reviews indicated that ESWT is well-tolerated and does not show a causal association with serious adverse events.

Even if the primary mechanism of action of Li-ESWT is believed to be the enhancement of tissue circulation through the stimulation of nitric oxide (NO) production, ESWT activates critical factors involved in connective tissue repair, such as fibroblasts, resulting in increased proliferation and expression of essential growth factors like TGF-beta-1 and collagen types I and III [18–22]. Although the evidence is still largely based on case studies, there are promising findings regarding the healing effects of ESWT following extensive tissue resection due to conditions such as Fournier's gangrene, demonstrating complete restoration of the affected local skin (e.g., perineal, penile, or scrotal areas) [23, 24] (**Figures 2** and **3**). The proposed underlying mechanism is the stimulation of stem cells, which has been experimentally validated in animal models related to pelvic floor trauma and erectile dysfunction [40, 41].

In summary, Li-ESWT shows considerable promise as a treatment modality for chronic wounds, with a favorable safety profile and potential mechanisms that support its efficacy in promoting wound healing and enhancing tissue repair.

The underlying mechanism of action for low-intensity extracorporeal shock wave therapy (Li-ESWT) is grounded in the concept of mechano-transduction [25]. This mechanism provides two key advantages:

1. Noninvasive mechanical force transmission: Extracorporeal shock waves serve as an excellent medium for delivering mechanical forces to nearly any cell in the human body in a noninvasive manner. This phenomenon is called mechano-transduction.

2. Low-intensity application of shock wave energy: Importantly, stimulation of mechano-transduction within cells does not require high-intensity levels, which minimizes the risk of adverse effects.

Recent clinical experiences with Li-ESWT have also demonstrated its efficacy in managing complex cases such as decubitus ulcers associated with fistulas. We observed that transcutaneous treatment of the infected area resulted in complete clearance, healing, and closure of both fistulas. This approach proved to be significantly more effective than traditional irrigation or vacuum application. After several weekly sessions, the purulent discharge ceased, transitioning to clear secretion before ultimately stopping altogether, resulting in the complete closure of the fistula (see **Figure 4**).

In this context, the re-epithelialization rate or re-epithelialization speed, as shown for three studies in **Table 6** [24, 34, 38], may be used as an objective parameter for future comparative studies evaluating the effect of LI-ESWT in the management of wound healing (**Figures 5** and **6**).

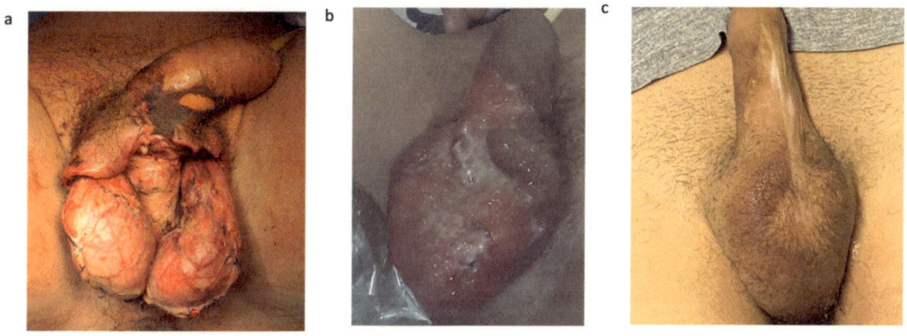

Figure 5.
Low-intensity extracorporeal shock wave therapy (Li-ESWT) using an electromagnetic device as a single management of wound healing following radical excision of infected tissue after Fournier's gangrene in a 32-year-old male patient. a) Radical excision of the involved tissue. b) Granulating tissue covering the wound after 6 weeks. c) Final cosmetic result after 6 months with complete restoration of penile and scrotal skin.

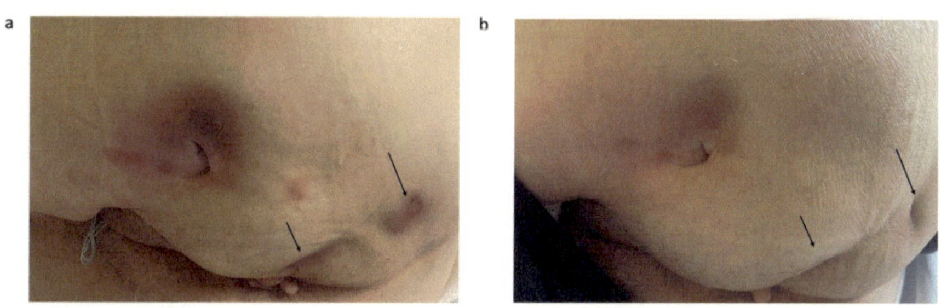

Figure 6.
Low-intensity extracorporeal shock wave therapy (Li-ESWT) using an electromagnetic device as a single management of wound healing of a decubitus with two fistulas in a 40-year-old female quadriplegic patient. a) Skin defect (3 × 4 cm) with two fistulas (arrows). b) Significant reduction of the skin defect after 9 months /2 × 2 cm) and complete healing of both fistulas.

Author	Lesion	Treatment groups	Wound area at day 0 (cm^2)	Wound area at end of treatment (cm^2)	Difference of wound area (cm^2)	Re-epithelization speed ($\Delta cm^2/d$)	Comment
Ottomann et al. [38]	Skin graft donor site of trauma patients	Defocused shock wave therapy 0.1 mJ/mm^2	n.a.	n.a.	n.a.	n.a.	Significantly faster healing of the donor site 13.9 versus 16.7 d
Dymarek R et al. [34]	Pressure ulcers Grade II and III	Radial ESWT (2 sessions)	13.5	7.3 (7 days)	6.2	0.9	Major skin cells, Keratinocytes, Fibroblasts are mechanosensitive
Rassweiler J et al. [24]	Fournier gangrene	Focused ESWT 0.25 mJ/mm^2 3–4 Hz, 2500 SW	18.7–99.7	0.0–55.3 (42–150 days)	10.1–99.9	0.24–0.79	Complete healing of the defect by local tissue (penile, scrotal, skin)

Table 6.
Comparison of re-epithelization effects and wound-healing rates in clinical studies (modified from Rassweiler et al. [24]).

Understanding Li-ESWT's efficacy and its theoretical basis will increase its potential as an advanced wound healing therapy. This chapter provides significant insights into how Li-ESWT may complement existing wound management strategies, thereby offering new options for patients with chronic wounds or ulcers.

11. Conclusions

This review highlights the potential of extracorporeal shock wave therapy as an advanced wound healing modality. The skin serves as an ideal platform to visualize healing progress and tissue restoration, providing a model for regenerative medicine.

The efficacy of ESWT, alongside its theoretical underpinnings, underscores its promise as a complementary approach to existing wound management strategies, offering new hope for patients with chronic wounds and ulcers. Thus, ESWT presents a compelling, noninvasive, and safe treatment option that can improve outcomes following extensive surgeries, such as those required for the management of Fournier's gangrene.

To optimize the benefits of ESWT in wound healing, further studies are necessary to standardize treatment protocols, encompassing factors such as shock wave intensity, frequency of impulses, and the number of treatment sessions required.

Conflict of interest

Prof. Jens Rassweiler is a consultant for Storz Medical, Taegerwilen, Switzerland. Prof. Wolfgang Schaden is a shareholder and International Medical Director of Tissue Regeneration Technologies, GA, USA, and Dr. Agatep and Dr. Condeno have no conflict of interest.

Author details

Jens J. Rassweiler[1*], Juvido Agatep[2], Clarice Condeno[2] and Wolfgang Schaden[3]

1 Department of Urology, University of Tübingen, Tübingen, Germany

2 Department of Urology, East Avenue Medical Center, Manila, Philippines

3 Ludwig Boltzmann Institute for Traumatology, Vienna, Austria

*Address all correspondence to: jens.rassweiler@gmail.com

References

[1] Chaussy C, Brendel W, Schmiedt E. Extracorporeally induced destruction of kidney stones by shock waves. Lancet. 1980;**2**:1265-1268

[2] Fuchs G, Miller K, Rassweiler J, Eisenberger F. Extracorporeal shock wave lithotripsy: One-year experience with the Dornier lithotripter. European Urology. 1985;**11**:145-149

[3] Abdel-Salam Y, Budair Z, Renner C, Frede T, Rassweiler J, El-Annany F, et al. Treatment of Peyronie's disease by extracorporeal shockwave therapy: Evaluation of our preliminary results. Journal of Endourology. 1999;**13**:549-552

[4] Rassweiler JJ, Scheitlin W, Goezen AS, Radecke F. Long-term experiences with high-energy shock wave therapy in the management chronic phase Peyronie's disease using two different electromagnetic lithotripters. World Journal of Urology. 2024;**42**(1):124. DOI: 10.1007/s00345-024-04792-x

[5] Haupt G, Haupt A, Ekkernkamp A, Gerety B, Chvapil M. Influence of shock waves on fracture healing. Urology. 1992;**39**(6):529-532. DOI: 10.1016/0090-4295(92)90009-l

[6] Rompe JD, Hopf C, Nafe B, Burger R. Low-energy extracorporeal shock wave therapy for painful heel: A prospective controlled single-blind study. Archives of Orthopaedic and Trauma Surgery. 1996;**115**:75-79

[7] Schaden W, Thiele R, Kölpl C, Pusch M, Nissan A, Attinger CE, et al. Shock wave therapy for acute and chronic soft tissue wounds: A feasibility study. The Journal of Surgical Research. 2007;**143**(1):1-12

[8] Knobloch K. ESWT an der Haut. In: DIGEST-Leitlinien. 2019. pp. 90-96. Available from: https://digestev.de/files/webpage/content/pdf/Leitlinien_Juni_2019.pdf [Accessed October 5, 2025]

[9] Haupt G, Haupt A, Ekkernkamp A, Gerety B, Chvapil M. Influence of shock wave healing. Urology. 1992;**39**:529-532

[10] Rassweiler J, Ringeisen M, Knobloch K, Schaden W. Efficacy and theoretical basis of low-intensity shock wave therapy in the management of different forms of wound healing: Own experiences and a review of the literature. Medical Research Archives. 2023;**11**(8):1-13. DOI: 10.18103/mra.v11i8.4394

[11] Aldana PC, Khachemoune A. Diabetic foot ulcers: Appraising standard of care and reviewing new trends in management. American Journal of Clinical Dermatology. 2020;**21**(2):255-264

[12] Norman G, Westby MJ, Rithalia AD, Stubbs N, Soares MO, Dumville JC. Dressings and topical agents for treating venous leg ulcers. Cochrane Database of Systematic Reviews. 2018;**15**(6):CD012583. DOI: 10.1002/14651858.CD012583

[13] Westby MJ, Dumville JC, Soares MO, Stubbs N, Norman G. Dressings and topical agents for treating pressure ulcers. Cochrane Database of Systematic Reviews. 2017;**22**(6):CD011947. DOI: 10.1002/14651858.CD011947

[14] Kranke P, Bennett MH, Martyn-St James M, Schnabel A, Debus SE, Weibel S. Hyperbaric oxygen therapy for chronic wounds.

Cochrane Database of Systematic Reviews. 2015;**24**(6):CD004123. DOI: 10.1002/14651858.CD004123

[15] Rassweiler JJ, Knoll T, Köhrmann KU, McAteer JA, Lingeman JE, Cleveland RO, et al. Shock wave technology and application – An update. European Urology. 2011;**59**:784-796

[16] Sramkova T, Motil I, Jarkovsky J, Sramkova K. Erectile dysfunction treatment using focused linear low-intensity extracorporeal shockwaves: Single-blind, sham-controlled, randomized clinical trial. Urologia Internationalis. 2020;**104**(5-6):417-424. DOI: 10.1159/000504788

[17] Dymarek R, Kuberka I, Rosińczuk J, Walewicz K, Taradaj J, Sopel M. The immediate clinical effects following a single radial shock wave therapy in pressure ulcers: A preliminary randomized controlled trial of the SHOWN project. Advances in Wound Care. 2023;**12**(8):440-452

[18] Mariotto SC, Amelio E, Ciampa AR, de Prati AC, Marlinghaus E, Russo S, et al. Extracorporeal shock waves: From lithotripsy to anti-inflammatory action by NO production. Nitric Oxide. 2005;**12**(2):89-96

[19] Kisch T, Wuerfel W, Forstmeier V, Liodaki E, Stang FH, Knobloch K, et al. Repetitive shock wave therapy improves muscular microcirculation. The Journal of Surgical Research. 2016;**201**(2):440-445

[20] Serizawa F, Ito K, Matsubara M, Sato A, Shimokawa H, Satomi S. Extracorporeal shock wave therapy induces therapeutic lymphangiogenesis in a rat model of secondary lymphoedema. European Journal of Vascular and Endovascular Surgery. 2011;**42**(2):254-260

[21] Mariotto SC, Cavalieri E, Amelio E, Marlinghaus E, Suzuki H. Extracorporeal shock wave therapy in inflammatory diseases: Molecular mechanism that triggers anti-inflammatory action. Current Medicinal Chemistry. 2009;**16**:2366-2372

[22] Frairia R, Berta L. Biological effects of extracorporeal shock waves on fibroblasts. A review. Muscles Ligaments Tendons Journal. 2011;**1**(4):138-147

[23] Rassweiler JJ, Scheitlin W, Goezen AS, Rassweiler-Seyfried MC. Low-energy shockwave therapy in the management of wound healing following Fournier's gangrene. European Urology Open Science. 2022;**45**:8-11

[24] Rassweiler JJ, Scheitlin W, Agatep J, Condeno C, Schaden W. Low-intensity extracorporeal shock wave therapy in the postoperative management of Fournier's gangrene-a case series of a new concept. Medical Research Archives. 2024;**12**(10):1-13. DOI: 10.18103/mra.v1210.5801

[25] Charras G, Yap AS. Tensile forces and mechanotransduction at cell-cell junctions. Current Biology. 2018;**28**:R445-R457

[26] Aguilera-Sáez J, Muñoz P, Serracanta J, Monte A, Barret JP. Extracorporeal shock wave therapy role in the treatment of burn patients. A systematic literature review. Burns. 2020;**46**(7):1525-1532

[27] Yang Y, Kang J, Jiang T, Schmitz C, Weng C, Zhang L. Safety and efficacy of treating post-burn pathological scars with extracorporeal shock wave therapy: A meta-analysis of randomized controlled trials. Wound Repair and Regeneration. 2022;**30**(5):595-607

[28] Omar MT, Gwada RF, Shaheen AA, Saggini R. Extracorporeal shockwave

therapy for the treatment of chronic wound of lower extremity: Current perspective and systematic review. International Wound Journal. 2017;**14**(6):898-908

[29] Hitchman LH, Totty JP, Raza A, Cai P, Smith GE, Carradice D, et al. Extracorporeal shockwave therapy for diabetic foot ulcers: A systematic review and meta-analysis. Annals of Vascular Surgery. 2019;**56**:330-339

[30] Huang Q, Yan P, Xiong H, Shuai T, Liu J, Zhu L, et al. Extracorporeal shock wave therapy for treating foot ulcers in adults with type 1 and type 2 diabetes: A systematic review and meta-analysis of randomized controlled trials. Canadian Journal of Diabetes. 2020;**44**(2):196-204.e3. DOI: 10.1016/j.jcjd.2019.05.006

[31] Hitchman L, Totty J, Smith GE, Carradice D, Twiddy M, Iglesias C, et al. Extracorporeal shockwave therapy compared with standard care for diabetic foot ulcer healing: An updated systematic review. International Wound Journal. 2023;**20**(6):2303-2320

[32] Zhang L, Weng C, Zhao Z, Fu X. Extracorporeal shock wave therapy for chronic wounds: A systematic review and meta-analysis of randomized controlled trials. Wound Repair and Regeneration. 2017;**25**(4):697-706

[33] Taheri P, Shahbandari M, Parvaresh M, Vahdatpour B. Extracorporeal shockwave therapy for chronic venous ulcers: A randomized controlled trial. Galen Medical Journal. 2021;**25**(10):e1931. DOI: 10.31661/gmj.v10i0.1931

[34] Dymarek R, Halski T, Ptaszkowski K, Slupska L, Rosinczuk J, Taradaj J. Extracorporeal shock wave therapy as an adjunct wound treatment: A systematic review of the literature. Ostomy/Wound Management. 2014;**60**(7):26-39

[35] Butterworth PA, Walsh TP, Pennisi YD, Chesne AD, Schmitz C, Nancarrow SA. The effectiveness of extracorporeal shock wave therapy for the treatment of lower limb ulceration: A systematic review. Journal of Foot and Ankle Research. 2015;**8**:3. DOI: 10.1186/s13047-014-0059-0

[36] Dolibog P, Franek A, Brzezińska-Wcisło L, Wróbel B, Arasiewicz H, Chmielewska D. Shockwave therapy in selected soft tissue diseases: A literature review. Journal of Wound Care. 2018;**27**(9):573-583

[37] Zhang L, Fu XB, Chen S, Zhao ZB, Schmitz C, Weng CS. Efficacy and safety of extracorporeal shock wave therapy for acute and chronic soft tissue wounds: A systematic review and meta-analysis. International Wound Journal. 2018;**15**(4):590-599

[38] Ottomann C, Hartmann B, Tyler J, Maier H, Thiele R, Schaden W, et al. Prospective randomized trial of accelerated re-epithelialization of skin graft donor sites using extracorporeal shock wave therapy. Journal of the American College of Surgeons. 2010;**211**(4):568-569. DOI: 10.1016/j.jamcollsurg.2010.08.008

[39] Chen J, Nie J. Effects of extracorporeal shock wave combined with vivaphototherapy on blood perfusion, inflammatory response, and prognosis in burn patients. Computational and Mathematical Methods in Medicine. 2022;**2022**(25):1386875. DOI: 10.1155/2022/1386875

[40] Lin G, Van Kuiken M, Wang G, Banie L, Tan Y, Zhou F, et al. Microenergy acoustic pulse therapy

restores function and structure of pelvic floor muscles after simulated birth injury. Translational Andrology and Urology. 2022;**11**(5):595-606

[41] Shin D, Jeon SH, Tian WJ, Kwon EB, Kim GE, Bae WJ, et al. Extracorporeal shock wave therapy combined with engineered mesenchymal stem cells expressing stromal cell-derived factor-1 can improve erectile dysfunction in streptozotocin-induced diabetic rats. Translational Andrology and Urology. 2021;**10**(6):2362-2372

Section 4

Advanced Strategies, Tissue Engineering and Future Directions

Chapter 6

Pharmacological and Biological Strategies as Regulators of Scarless Wound Healing and Regeneration of Skin

Zhifeng Liao, Xi Chen, Nathalie Hirt-Burri, Alexandre Porcello, Cíntia Marques, Kelly Lourenço, Alexis Laurent and Lee Ann Applegate

Abstract

Adult human skin typically repairs deep wounds by forming scar tissue, a process that often results in compromised function and aesthetics. In stark contrast, observations of human fetal skin *in utero*, up to certain gestational stages, demonstrate a remarkable capacity for true tissue regeneration, characterized by rapid healing and the complete absence of scar formation. This chapter explore into the specific cellular factors and their interplay with the extracellular matrix (ECM) that orchestrate this exceptional regenerative process, including multiple individual growth factors (GFs) (EGF, TGF-β, PDGF, FGF, IGF) and other collagen metabolism/deposition factors and inhibitors. Furthermore, we will discuss the distinctions between these relatively traditional pharmacological approaches of the application of growth factors and cytokines and cutting-edge innovative biological medicines, particularly cellular therapies. Looking at specific cell sources and cell therapies, we will examine elements and formulations collectively for their role in remodeling and functional restoration of skin tissue, which is similar to that seen in fetal wound healing. This comparative analysis will highlight their respective roles and potential in achieving anti-fibrotic and anti-scar effects in human skin, drawing insights from the unparalleled example of fetal regeneration.

Keywords: fetal skin, extracellular matrix, fibroblasts, collagen, scar-free, regenerative medicine, growth factors, cytokines, cell therapy

1. Introduction to classical wound healing phases

Wound healing, a fundamental biological process essential for tissue repair and integrity, represents a highly dynamic and exquisitely complex cascade involving a myriad of cell types. These cells orchestrate an extensive array of biological events and intricate intercellular and tissue interactions, progressing through a series of sequential and tightly coordinated phases. Irrespective of the wound's etiology or chronicity, the healing process is conventionally divided into four overlapping yet distinct stages: (1) hemostasis, (2) inflammation, (3) proliferation, and (4) remodeling (**Figure 1**) [1].

The initial phase, hemostasis, is the body's immediate response to vascular injury, designed to limit blood loss and establish a provisional matrix for subsequent repair.

Following hemostasis, the inflammatory phase commences, characterized by a carefully orchestrated influx of immune cells and accompanied by crucial elimination of cellular debris, bacteria, and other potential pathogens, which promotes tissue debridement and signals the transition to the proliferative phase.

The third phase, proliferation, marks the beginning of tissue regeneration and wound closure and a shift toward an anti-inflammatory cytokine profile, fostering an environment conducive to tissue growth.

Finally, the remodeling phase is the longest and most critical for achieving functional and structural integrity, with the outcome of this phase dictating the final quality of the scar, ranging from a barely perceptible mark to hypertrophic or keloid scarring, reflecting the intricate balance of pro-fibrotic and anti-fibrotic signals [1].

Each phase of wound healing presents distinct opportunities for intervention, with specific physical actions and therapies tailored to the wound's etiology. For instance, in chronic wounds characterized by high fibrin content and necrotic tissue, effective debridement—either physically through methods like negative pressure wound therapy (NPWT) or curettage, or enzymatically—is crucial to initiate the subsequent healing phases. While general wound management principles such as debridement, cleaning, and antimicrobial treatment with appropriate dressings remain consistent across many wound types, significant advancements have been made in optimizing each stage of this intricate process.

The growing prevalence of chronic wounds and their associated complications, such as persistent infection, poses a substantial burden on healthcare systems and significantly diminishes patients' quality of life. The increasing incidence of comorbidities, including diabetes, obesity, malnutrition, and the global aging population, further exacerbates this challenge. This escalating healthcare demand has spurred the development of a diverse array of therapeutic approaches designed to optimize wound care at every stage.

Innovations span a wide spectrum, starting with enhanced instrument-based therapies like hyperbaric oxygen therapy (HBOT) and low-level laser therapy (LLLT), which aim to improve tissue perfusion and cellular activity. Advancements in wound dressings include novel antimicrobial materials and biologically active components such as hyaluronic acid (HA) and collagen, which provide a supportive environment for healing. Pharmaceutical interventions continue to evolve with the targeted application of cytokines and growth factors to modulate cellular responses. Furthermore, the field of biological medicines, particularly cellular therapies, holds immense promise for promoting regeneration.

A key emphasis is now placed on early-stage wound management, particularly in the realm of debridement. Here, intriguing innovations are emerging, such as the development of biologically mimetic enzymes. These include recombinant enzymes inspired by the highly effective, pain-free debridement mechanisms observed in medical maggot therapy, offering a new frontier in wound bed preparation [2].

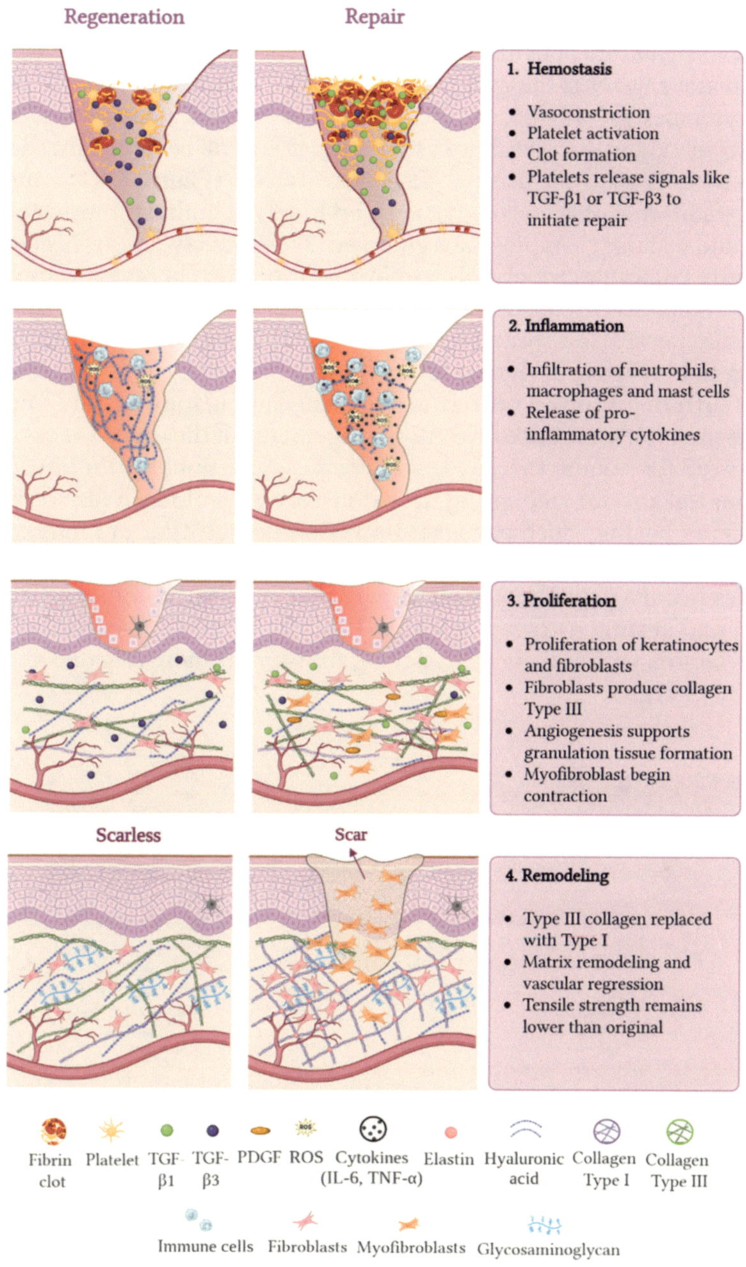

Figure 1.
Stages of wound healing, including hemostasis, inflammation, proliferation, and remodeling, and their major factors implicated during the complex process, with associated differences between scarless and scar formation, which depend on repair vs. regenerative processes. Wound healing begins with the hemostasis phase (1) involving vasoconstriction, platelet activation, clot formation, and final release from platelets of factors initiating repair processes (TGF-β1 increased in repair and TGF-β3 increased for regeneration). This phase leads into the inflammation (2) with neutrophil, macrophage, and mast cell infiltration and the release of pro-inflammatory cytokines. Proliferation phase, (3) is initiated by cellular proliferation of keratinocytes and fibroblasts associated with cellular production of collagen Type III by fibroblasts. Angiogenesis supporting granulation tissue formation arises, and myofibroblast contraction is initiated (higher myofibroblasts in repair). Remodeling (4) of tissue begins with Type III collagen replacing Type I (Type III collagen increased in repair and Type I collagen increased in regeneration) and matrix remodeling with vascular regression, with associated tensile strength decreasing (tensile strength decreased in repair).

Each distinct phase of wound healing, once wounds are appropriately debrided, offers critical insights into potential therapeutic targets, particularly for developing anti-inflammatory agents to mitigate persistent pro-inflammatory states. To this end, numerous cytokines, growth factors, and enzymes have been extensively investigated for their capacity to modulate the healing cascade, and these will be thoroughly described in the initial section focusing on pharmacological treatments (**Figure 2**, left column).

Beyond traditional pharmacology, new and highly promising approaches utilizing biologicals and cellular therapies have emerged. These involve diverse cellular sources and innovative combinations of cells and formulations for therapeutic application. A significant emphasis in this chapter will be placed on those therapies specifically aimed at achieving scarless wound healing and on the most recent advancements in this exciting field (**Figure 2**, right column).

Patients suffering from severe burns represent a population acutely concerned with long-term outcomes related to scar management. In these critical cases, the immediate need for cellular therapy is often paramount, not only for life-saving interventions but also for facilitating the extensive and prolonged recovery inherent in severe wound healing. Such scenarios necessitate a multitude of innovative measures to ensure the optimal quality of life for the patient. Decades of experience with cell therapies in burn patients have illuminated the specific cell types pivotal in the complex wound healing pathway, as well as the critical roles of particular cytokines and growth factors within these cells, paving the way for more targeted and effective regenerative strategies.

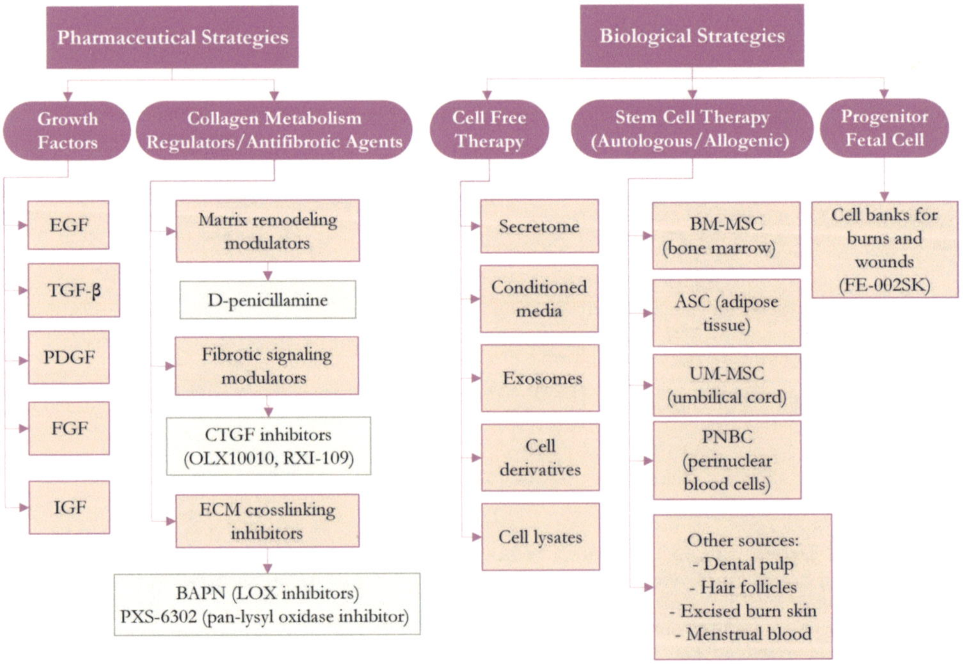

Figure 2.
Pharmaceutical and biological strategies for scarless wound healing. Pharmaceutical strategies concentrate on single or combined growth factors involved in collagen metabolism and antifibrotic processes. Biological strategies vary from progenitor (fetal cell therapy) and stem cells, which may be autologous or allogenic (derived from bone marrow, adipose, umbilical, blood cells, hair follicles, etc.), to cell-free strategies including secretome, exosomes, and cell lysates.

1.1 Fetal wound healing

It had been documented already in the 1970s that early human fetal skin could heal without scar formation. This was found to be tissue-specific and also related to the developmental age [3]. The remarkable capacity for scarless wound healing observed in fetal skin stands in stark contrast to the typical fibrotic repair mechanisms in adults, offering crucial insights into regenerative biology. Several prominent differences underpin this disparity. Fetal tissue repair is characterized by a significantly attenuated inflammatory reaction compared to adult healing. Furthermore, fetal wounds exhibit substantial deposition of glycosaminoglycans (GAGs), particularly hyaluronic acid (HA). HA is recognized for its critical roles in facilitating cellular migration and proliferation, which are essential processes during effective wound repair (**Figure 1**, first column—regeneration/scarless).

Beyond the unique extracellular matrix composition, fetal wounds demonstrate a notably lower degree of collagen organization, a characteristic potentially linked to their scarless outcome. Investigations into growth factor profiles reveal further distinctions. Platelet-Derived Growth Factor (PDGF) is consistently present within fetal wounds. However, it has been observed that Transforming Growth Factor-beta (TGF-β) and basic Fibroblast Growth Factor (bFGF) are not present. The absence of these latter factors may contribute significantly to the limited neovascularization and reduced collagen deposition typically seen in fetal wounds.

Given that platelets and macrophages are well-established sources of TGF-β in adult wound healing, the observed lack of TGF-β in fetal wounds could be directly related to less pronounced platelet degranulation and a diminished infiltration of macrophages into the fetal wound site. In turn, the attenuated presence of TGF-β is strongly implicated in the overall decreased inflammatory response characteristic of fetal scarless healing. These distinctive molecular and cellular environments provide compelling targets for future regenerative strategies. Early studies using injections into the wound with growth factors in rats support these proposed mechanistic pathways [4].

Rapidly during the 1990s, intense research began with different models using human skin. Compelling experimental evidence by Lorenz et al. [5] further underscores that the capacity for scarless wound healing is an intrinsic property of fetal skin, rather than being solely dependent on the *in utero* environment. Early studies, utilizing xenograft models, demonstrated that human fetal skin samples, when transplanted onto nude mice and subsequently incised, consistently healed with a scarless phenotype. This seminal finding provided initial support for the autonomous regenerative potential of fetal tissue.

Further sophisticated investigations by the same research group bolstered this hypothesis. In a remarkable experiment, adult sheepskin was heterotopically transplanted onto the dorsum of a fetal sheep *in utero*. Upon wounding, the adult skin graft healed with characteristic fibrosis at the incision sites, contrasting sharply with the scarless repair observed in the surrounding fetal tissue. These pivotal results conclusively demonstrated that the scarless wound healing phenomenon in the fetus is primarily attributable to intrinsic cellular functions and the unique characteristics of fetal dermal components, rather than being dictated by external factors such as amniotic fluid composition or the generalized uterine environment. This body of work has been fundamental in directing research toward understanding the cellular and molecular underpinnings of fetal regeneration. Furthermore, these *in situ* experiments might also suggest that amniotic fluid itself is not potent enough to stimulate regeneration/repair of wounds [6–8]. An additional model was used in the early 1990s by Armstrong and Ferguson [9] with the fetal model of *Monodelphis domestica* (South American opossum). Further compelling evidence supporting the intrinsic nature of scarless healing and its gestational timing comes from this unique animal model. This marsupial presents an unusual developmental feature: its embryos are external from day one postconception, developing without the protective confines of a pouch or direct contact with amniotic fluid. This unique *ex utero* development provides an unparalleled opportunity to study early embryonic wound healing in a more accessible manner.

Experimental studies on the skin of these marsupial embryos have revealed striking parallels to human fetal development. Specifically, wounds inflicted on early gestation *Monodelphis d.* embryos (a developmental stage comparable to the first trimester in humans) consistently healed with no scar formation. In contrast, later gestation *Monodelphis d.* fetuses (analogous to the second and third trimesters in human development) demonstrated fibrotic scar formation following wounding, a response similar to that observed in adult marsupials.

These findings from the M*onodelphis d.* model strongly corroborate the concept that the capacity for scarless healing is an intrinsic, developmentally regulated property of early embryonic skin. Moreover, they reinforce the idea of a critical developmental window during which this regenerative ability is lost, transitioning to a scar-forming phenotype. This comparative biological insight further emphasizes the cellular and molecular mechanisms inherent to the developing organism, independent of a typical intrauterine environment, which govern the intricate processes of wound repair and regeneration.

Collectively, evidence from diverse mammalian models underscores that the early mammalian fetus exhibits remarkable regenerative processes in response to injury. Unlike adult wound repair, fetal healing leads to a complete restoration of normal skin architecture, characterized by an absence of significant inflammation, minimal or no contraction of surrounding tissue, and, crucially, the lack of scar formation. This unparalleled capacity for regeneration, rather than fibrotic repair, makes fetal wound healing a compelling model for understanding the mechanisms underlying true tissue restoration.

The fundamental differences between fetal and postnatal wound healing have been the subject of extensive investigation, delving into disparities at both the molecular and protein expression levels. Increasingly, recent data highlight that a key overarching mechanism governing this scarless phenomenon is intrinsically linked to the unique composition and dynamic regulation of extracellular matrix (ECM) components. Understanding how the fetal ECM environment supports regenerative outcomes, in contrast to the fibrogenic environment of adult wounds, is paramount for developing novel therapeutic strategies aimed at promoting scarless healing in a postnatal context [10, 11].

Despite significant advancements in identifying numerous individual proteins and molecular pathways implicated in scarless wound healing, translating these discoveries into effective clinical therapies has presented considerable challenges. To date, most therapeutic developments in this domain have yielded limited major progress in achieving truly scar-free outcomes in adult skin.

Nevertheless, clinical research has intensified considerably in recent years, driven by a burgeoning interest in aesthetic medicine, advanced skin care, and the broader pursuit of regenerative approaches. This heightened focus has led to a proliferation of novel therapeutic propositions. These include new cytokines and growth factors, often investigated in various synergistic combinations, specifically targeted at enhancing skin homeostasis, achieving antiaging effects, and, critically, promoting scar-free tissue repair and regeneration. The ongoing push for innovative solutions reflects both the unmet clinical need for improved scar management and the growing understanding of the intricate biological processes that govern tissue repair and regeneration.

2. Pharmaceutical strategies of scarless wound healing

2.1 Growth factors (EGF, TGF-β, PDGF, FGF, IGF)

Growth factors (GFs) are fundamental polypeptides that orchestrate crucial cellular processes by binding to specific receptors on target cell surfaces (**Figure 2**, left column). These potent signaling molecules regulate cell proliferation, metabolism, and differentiation, exerting a powerful influence on the intricate pathways of wound healing and tissue repair, even when present in minute, nanogram quantities. Growth factors are often classified based on various characteristics:

1. Target cell recognition: For example, Epidermal Growth Factor (EGF) primarily acts on epidermal cells, stimulating their synthetic and mitogenic activity, while Fibroblast Growth Factor (FGF) similarly targets fibroblasts.

2. Origin or source: Platelet-Derived Growth Factor (PDGF), for instance, is predominantly released from platelets. Similarly, Transforming Growth Factors (TGFs) can originate from various transformed cells.

3. Structural or functional homology: Insulin-like Growth Factors (IGFs) derive their name from their structural and biological similarities to insulin.

Growth factors exert their effects through diverse modes of action: they can act locally on the cells that produce them (autocrine function), on adjacent cells (paracrine function), within the producing cell itself (intracrine function), or even on distant cells through systemic circulation (endocrine secretion).

For effective tissue regeneration, growth factors involved in wound healing must be delivered to the wound site in a manner that ensures their bioactivity. However, the direct, single application of growth factors has often proven ineffective. This limited efficacy stems from several challenges: the hostile wound microenvironment, which can degrade GFs; diminished activity and poor tissue penetration; and the necessity for sustainable release and effective receptor binding.

Consequently, extensive research has focused on developing sophisticated delivery systems, advanced biomaterials, and strategies for modulating these molecules to achieve prolonged drug bioactivity and enable the use of lower, sustained doses. This approach aims to minimize the need for repeat exposures and reduce undesirable off-target effects. Key growth factors studied in wound healing include, but are not limited to, Epidermal Growth Factor (EGF), Transforming Growth Factor-beta (TGF-β), Platelet-Derived Growth Factor (PDGF), Fibroblast Growth Factor (FGF), and Insulin-like Growth Factor (IGF).

While some of these specific growth factors have demonstrated limited clinical relevance when administered individually, more recent evidence strongly suggests that combinations of growth factors can elicit superior synergistic effects, leading to greater overall efficacy. This aligns with the natural complexity of wound healing, which never relies on a single molecule but rather involves a highly orchestrated interplay of diverse components across different stages. Therefore, research efforts are increasingly focused on utilizing combinations of different growth factors designed to interact at specific phases of healing; for example, combining EGF to promote fibroblast migration with bFGF to enhance collagen deposition, thereby achieving a multifaceted therapeutic effect [12].

The development of sophisticated delivery systems is crucial for harnessing the full therapeutic potential of growth factors (GFs) in wound healing. Recent advancements have focused on creating composite cryogel systems designed for the sequential release of multiple GF groups, mimicking the natural, dynamic cascade of healing.

A notable example comes from the work of Jimi *et al.*, who engineered a novel chitosan-based cryogel. This system was specifically designed to deliver growth factors in a staged manner in murine wound models. Initially, the cryogel released Interleukin-10 (IL-10) and Transforming Growth Factor-beta (TGF-β), acting as inflammation modulatory factors. This was followed by the subsequent release of Vascular Endothelial Growth Factor (VEGF) and basic Fibroblast Growth Factor (bFGF), intended to promote later phases of wound healing, including neovascularization, wound closure, granulation tissue formation, and epithelialization.

Their research demonstrated that this chitosan-based gel provided controlled release of the growth factors while maintaining their biological activity and stability. Crucially, the sequential delivery strategy—first anti-inflammatory/modulatory factors, then pro-healing factors—resulted in superior overall wound healing outcomes in the mouse model. This approach highlights the importance of not just delivering growth factors but precisely controlling their timing and sequence to optimize the complex biological processes of wound repair [13].

2.1.1 Epidermal growth factor (EGF)

The seminal discovery of Epidermal Growth Factor (EGF) in the 1960s revolutionized research into growth factors (GFs) and cytokines. The subsequent decades yielded a wealth of information regarding their intricate involvement in disease pathophysiology and, crucially, their reparative mechanisms in wound healing [14].

EGF is a small 53-amino acid polypeptide primarily known for its role in stimulating epithelial cells. While it can also stimulate fibroblasts and smooth muscle cells, among others, its initial recognition stemmed from its capacity to promote keratinocyte migration and proliferation along wound beds. Early research also highlighted EGF's marked ability to accelerate development in neonatal and juvenile mice, underscoring its broader importance in organismal development [15]. These compelling regenerative observations prompted numerous clinical investigations into EGF's therapeutic potential.

Early clinical trials, for instance, combined topical EGF with silver sulfadiazine for donor sites in 12 burn or reconstructive surgery patients. While a statistically significant, albeit marginal, difference in healing time (1 day) was observed compared to silver sulfadiazine alone, the study noted high variability in overall healing; three patients showed early healing by day 4, while nine experienced delayed healing up to 20 days [16]. This initial prospective study, showcasing some effect with a single GF, paved the way for further investigations in chronic wounds, abdominal incisions, and burns. A trend emerged suggesting that topical EGF (10 μg/gm cream, twice daily) could improve healing in recalcitrant wounds, with closure times ranging from 12 to 92 days, though one of nine patients failed to respond [17]. Similarly, recombinant human EGF (rh-EGF) was subsequently used in the treatment of chronic ulcers, showing a tendency toward greater ulcer size reduction and improved overall healing, though results were not statistically different from controls. Notably, rh-EGF demonstrated a favorable safety profile with no reported side effects, and while a significant enhancement of re-epithelialization in venous ulcers was not observed, a 7% reduction in ulcer size compared to 3% with placebo was encouraging [18].

The relatively modest impact of these early clinical trials can be attributed to several factors. The use of silver sulfadiazine as a vehicle, for instance, was not entirely neutral. Moreover, the dosages of EGF employed in these trials may have been insufficient to elicit significant clinical efficacy. Crucially, it became evident that EGF likely requires sustained-release delivery for optimal effect.

This latter hypothesis was elegantly explored and clinically validated by Professor Jorge Berlanga-Acosta's clinical group in Cuba. Over much of his career, Professor Berlanga-Acosta has dedicated his efforts to optimizing EGF delivery, particularly to prevent amputations in diabetic foot ulcer patients [19]. His group's extensive pharmacovigilance and basic studies convincingly demonstrated the significance of local infiltration of growth factors for chronic wound healing. They further established that prolonged local bioavailability and continuous interaction with EGF receptors are essential for a successful tissue response. This understanding prompted a shift from topical EGF formulations to optimized injectable EGF for local infiltration into diabetic ulcers, thereby circumventing the limitations of topical applications and protecting the growth factor from the hostile microenvironment of chronic wounds, thus enhancing its bioavailability.

In retrospect, the initial EGF clinical work appeared somewhat premature concerning the fundamental scientific understanding of its molecular pharmacology, as pioneered by Davidson's group in 1985 [20]. Davidson's work had unequivocally demonstrated that EGF's efficacy in mouse wound healing models was directly tied to prolonged, sustained, and slow-release formulations, requiring at least 8–12 hours of continuous receptor stimulation to elicit a mitogenic signal. Such formulations dramatically increased fibroblast proliferation, secretion, and matrix deposition/organization.

Integrating these fundamental insights with prior clinical observations, Berlanga-Acosta formulated a clinical protocol for a compassionate use study in 2001, employing injections of EGF directly into the wound base and margins of terminal ulcers. This approach aimed to achieve a higher pharmacodynamic response, leading to enhanced granulation tissue growth and wound closure. In this study, 25 μg of EGF was applied three times weekly for 8 weeks, and remarkably, amputation was prevented in 58.6% of the 29 patients [21]. A subsequent randomized controlled study compared two different doses of rhEGF injections (75 or 25 μg, three times weekly for 8 weeks) directly into wounds. This study provided compelling evidence that the higher dose was well-tolerated and could significantly increase wound healing in patients [22]. These studies have, indeed, provided the necessary efficacy data to establish clinical pathways for international groups, who have subsequently adopted this delivery route to achieve higher wound healing rates and, critically, significantly lower amputation rates in diabetic patients.

Further groups implementing this protocol have reported similar successes. For instance, a Mexican cohort demonstrated that intralesional application of rhEGF at 75 μg, three times weekly, resulted in more complete ulcer healing and decreased ulcer size compared to placebo at 8 weeks. This underscores that rhEGF intralesional application can lead to improved patient outcomes, restoring normal foot function and enhancing the quality of life for individuals with diabetic foot ulcers [23]. While some transient side effects, including dizziness, localized pain and burning upon application, chills, and tremors, were noted, these are often outweighed by the severe impact of amputations in diabetic patients, which are common, complex, and carry a high economic burden.

Taken together, these collective studies emphatically demonstrate that formulation and administration are critically important factors when utilizing single growth factors in a clinical setting.

2.1.2 Transforming growth factor-beta (TGF-β)

Members of the Transforming Growth Factor-beta (TGF-β) family are recognized as crucial mediators in fundamental biological processes, including embryogenesis, tissue repair, oncogenesis, and fibrosis. The differential expression and relative ratios of various isoforms of TGF-β were initially considered central to the phenomenon of scarless healing observed in the fetus, making them a primary focus of research interest.

From a pharmaceutical standpoint, early efforts to achieve scarless wound healing and effective scar management largely targeted Transforming Growth Factor-beta (TGF-β) itself. This growth factor, along with its isoforms (TGF-β1, TGF-β2, and TGF-β3), is secreted by a variety of cell types at injury sites, including platelets, fibroblasts, and macrophages. TGF-β is a major orchestrator of inflammatory cell migration, extracellular matrix (ECM) synthesis, and matrix turnover. It was hypothesized that the ratio of these isoforms plays a critical role in scarless wound healing, given that fetal skin typically exhibits higher levels of TGF-β3 compared to adult skin. However, our own investigations into isoform ratios in cultured human fetal skin cells revealed a different picture: TGF-β1 gene expression was significantly higher than the other two isoforms, with a very high TGF-β1 to TGF-β3 ratio of 21.47 ± 1.98 [24].

Clinical trials involving recombinant TGF-β3 (Avotermin/Juvista®) initially showed promise in Phase I and II studies for scar management. However, this product failed to meet its primary and secondary endpoints in a subsequent Phase III trial. Consequently, the commercialization agreement between Shire and Renovo (a Manchester, England-based company), valued at £825 million, was terminated following the unsuccessful Phase III trial in 2011.

Another injectable product, mannose-6-phosphate (M6P), marketed as Juvidex® by the same company, was also tested pre-clinically and clinically. This product was designed to reduce scar formation by binding TGF-β to the M6P/IGF-2 receptor, which in turn converts latent TGF-β to its active form and was subsequently thought to decrease the levels of active TGF-β isoforms 1 and 2. Despite its hypothesized mechanism, Juvidex® also failed to meet its primary endpoints in a Phase II placebo-controlled trial designed to accelerate skin graft donor site healing. Furthermore, a different formulation of M6P at high doses (Adaprev®, 600 mM M6P) was tested pre-clinically in mouse and rabbit models for its anti-fibrotic effects on tendons [25], but it too did not demonstrate significant overall improvements.

The characteristic absence of robust inflammation in scarless wound healing also prompted investigations into the roles of various interleukins involved in pro- and anti-inflammatory processes. Interleukin-10 (IL-10), in particular, was further developed for human anti-scarring trials by the same company (Renovo) that investigated

TGF-β and M6P, under the name Prevascar®. However, a Phase III study involving an African American cohort of 56 patients revealed no significant differences in scar management outcomes for incisions treated with Prevascar®.

The collective experiences with individual growth factors and cytokines highlight the profound complexity of modulating wound healing toward a scarless architecture and underscore the inherent difficulties in translating findings from animal models to successful human clinical trials. Renovo, the company behind these five products (Juvista – rhTGF-β3 for anti-scar; Adaprev – M6P for anti-scar/fibrosis in tendons; Prevascar – IL-10 for anti-scar *via* suppression of TGF-β1 and TGF-β2; Juvidex – lower dose M6P as a cosmetic ingredient; and RN1005 – targeting the Wnt pathway for scar reduction and tissue regeneration) at different phases of development, ultimately halted all its clinical pharmaceutical development. The company subsequently transitioned to become a financial provider several years later under the name Inspired Capital plc, having become a cash-shell company with £30 million [25–32].

2.1.3 Platelet-derived growth factor (PDGF)

Platelet-Derived Growth Factor (PDGF) is a crucial mitogen derived primarily from platelets during blood coagulation, making it a central component of the complex wound healing cascade. As a potent chemoattractant for neutrophils, PDGF acts as an important inflammatory mediator, initiating early events in wound repair. Beyond its role in inflammation, PDGF also functions as a powerful chemoattractant for fibroblasts and a stimulator of both collagen synthesis and collagenase activity, processes intricately involved in extracellular matrix (ECM) remodeling during healing. Furthermore, PDGF engages in complex interactions with other growth factors, including inhibiting EGF binding to its receptor, stimulating IGF-I production, and mediating the mitogenic effects of TGF-β on fibroblasts [33].

Notably, Becaplermin (Regranex®, Smith & Nephew) represents one of the few single growth factor-based medications developed for clinical use, specifically investigated for chronic ulcerations such as diabetic foot ulcers and pressure ulcers. Introduced in 2001, this 0.01% (100 μg/mL) recombinant human PDGF-BB (rhPDGF-BB) was a significant advancement in wound and scar management. Its primary mode of action is to promote cutaneous wound healing by modulating dermal fibroblast proliferation and migration, stimulating ECM deposition, and attracting other essential cells (e.g., neutrophils, monocytes, and smooth muscle cells) to the wound bed, thereby fostering tissue repair and healthy collagen production. Topical application of rhPDGF-BB has been shown to primarily enhance wound healing through the robust formation of granulation tissue, increased ECM synthesis, and modulation of the inflammatory phase of the wound healing process [34]. Although an early "black box warning" was issued by the FDA due to potential side effects, this was later lifted years later [35, 36]. However, its use in Europe was discontinued in 2011 [37].

In the context of fetal wound healing, PDGF gene expression has been shown to be higher in early fetal skin compared to later developmental stages, without significant overall alterations in fibroblast populations. However, PDGF is well-known to actively recruit fibroblasts and accelerate ECM deposition. Early studies utilizing fetal rabbits demonstrated that the exogenous addition of PDGF to skin resulted in significant local inflammation, pronounced fibroblast recruitment, and increased collagen and hyaluronic acid deposition at the implant site. Importantly, this response was both dose-dependent and contingent on the duration of PDGF presence, with effective concentrations ranging from 1 to 10 ng of active substance [38]. The pro-fibrotic reactivity observed in fetal skin exposed to exogenous PDGF strongly suggests that natural scarless fetal repair likely proceeds in the absence or with a significantly diminished presence of PDGF. Indeed, mechanistic studies in rat fibroblasts have shown that the expression of the PDGF-β receptor is lower in fetal fibroblasts compared to adult fibroblasts, further supporting the *in vivo* rabbit model data [39]. Overall, it is increasingly clear that no single factor is solely responsible for scarless wound healing; rather, a precise and dynamic balance of multiple interacting factors is essential for achieving such a regenerative outcome.

2.1.4 Fibroblast growth factor (FGF)

The Fibroblast Growth Factor (FGF) family comprises 23 distinct members, with FGF-2 (basic FGF, bFGF), FGF-7 (Keratinocyte Growth Factor-1, KGF-1), FGF-9, and FGF-10 (KGF-2) being among the most extensively characterized. bFGF, in particular, has a well-established role in promoting angiogenesis, stimulating the migration of fibroblasts and macrophages, and facilitating re-epithelialization.

Early clinical studies investigated bFGF in pressure ulcers, using low (100 mg/L), intermediate (500 mg/L), and high (1 g/L) doses [40]. When all the combined data from the treated groups were compared to the control, a slightly better performance for overall wound closure was observed in the treated groups, showing a 69% decrease in wound volume for bFGF-treated wounds compared to 59% for the placebo. While blinded observers could distinguish between treated ulcers, no major dose dependency was evident, likely due to the small number of patients per subgroup. These early clinical findings spurred further research into optimizing formulations for growth factors within this family.

Other FGF family members, such as FGF-7, have also been developed for clinical use in various mucosal tissue repairs, demonstrating improved wound healing responses [41]. However, further development of FGFs, including Repifermin (KGF-2), was terminated in 2004 due to failed clinical trials for mucosal ulceration [42]. This rapid trajectory of development and subsequent termination, similar to that observed with the EGF family, underscores the complexities of translating growth factor research into successful clinical products. Past clinical experiences strongly suggest that greater attention to dose, delivery, and formulation could significantly impact the efficacy of treatment regimens for many growth factors involved in wound repair.

More recent interest in FGFs has been fueled by findings that different FGFs are expressed at higher levels in early human fetal fibroblasts compared to those from later gestation, aligning with the period when scarless wound healing is observed [43]. While animal studies on FGFs in fetal wounds sometimes present contradictory results, FGFs are generally known to stimulate cellular migration, proliferation, fibroblast activation, and angiogenesis. However, similar to other GFs, the therapeutic effect of FGF administration to wounds appears to depend critically on the specific isoform, its formulation, and the administration method.

FGF-2, which was notably upregulated in early human fetal fibroblasts, has been utilized in topical formulations for chronic wounds and pressure sores. Its recombinant form, Trafermin, was employed by Olympus Biotech Corporation in diabetic chronic foot ulcers, demonstrating higher rates of wound healing in the Trafermin-treated patient group. A large European study, divided into Northern and Southern regions, involving 369 patients treated with a 0.01% Trafermin spray, showed a relative wound regression of 40% at 6 weeks, with approximately 61% wound closure in the Trafermin group versus 53% in the placebo group [44, 45].

Although bFGF may not yet have widespread international recognition for wound and scar management, a recent Japanese review of their 20-year clinical experience with this growth factor provided valuable insights [46]. Based on seven case reports, four clinical studies, and five randomized controlled trials, the consensus was that further research and broader recognition are needed for bFGF to fully exploit its clinical advantages. Moreover, increased emphasis has been placed on the controlled release of bFGF, similar to other growth factors, as this has shown better healing outcomes in mouse full-thickness wound models [47]. It has been suggested that alternative formulations could not only provide greater convenience but also improve wound healing and further reduce the risk of postsurgical scar formation.

Indeed, Japan has a unique and extensive clinical experience with bFGF, as recombinant human bFGF (rhbFGF) has been registered since 2001 as the world's first rhbFGF preparation marketed in Japan as a topical spray for accelerating the healing of burn wounds and diabetic leg ulcers (Fiblast®, Kaken Pharmaceutical Co., Tokyo, Japan). With significant clinical experience and a good safety profile, Fiblast® was even included in the Clinical Practice Guidelines for Burn Injuries by the Japanese Society for Burns in 2009 for second-degree burns [46]. Furthermore, Kaken Pharmaceutical registered Regroth® in 2016 for periodontal regeneration.

bFGF has also shown effective treatment in wound repair and scar prevention in pediatric second- to third-degree burns. While a limited group of 20 patients did not allow for statistically significant differences in wound closure rates (17.9 days for bFGF vs. 19.6 days for control), overall better healing, scar appearance, color, and wound quality at one year showed encouraging results [48]. In a subsequent study for pediatric palmar burns, it was demonstrated that early administration of bFGF could prevent scar contracture when skin grafting was not necessary, and better pigmentation was observed during follow-up [49].

Interestingly, FGF-2 was already approved in China and Japan for chronic wounds, pressure sores, and skin ulcers [50]. It has been used clinically in China for several decades, including recombinant bovine bFGF (rbFGF-Torita Bio-Pharmaceutical Industry Co., Zhuhai, China) [51] and recombinant human acidic FGF (rh-aFGF) (WanXing Biology Pharmaceuticals Company, Shanghai, China). While clinical trials with rh-aFGF showed a statistically significant, albeit small, difference in healing time for donor site wounds or burns, a double-blind, randomized, and placebo-controlled study reported mean healed times of 17.23 vs. 18.92 days for rh-aFGF vs. placebo for burns and 13.07 vs. 14.71 days for donor sites, respectively. While safety was reported, the authors recognized the need for long-term follow-up before extensive clinical use [52].

Since the 1980s, both the US Wound Healing Society and the European Wound Management Association have recommended FGF for refractory wounds. Within the FGF family, FGF-2 and FGF-10 have been particularly emphasized for cutaneous wound healing. This led Kaken Pharmaceutical Co. to acquire the recombinant bacterial strain expressing human FGF-2 (Trafermin) and associated patents from Johnson & Johnson in the United States. Following more than a decade of research, Kaken successfully registered Fiblast® for pressure sores and skin ulcers (including both burn ulcers and foot ulcers), as described above.

Overall, among other mechanisms, bFGF may help prevent excessive dermal collagen deposition and aid in the appropriate development of the extracellular matrix within the wound. This is in addition to its known roles in promoting fibroblast proliferation, enhancing fibroblast migration, and inhibiting their differentiation into myofibroblasts, thereby contributing to the prevention of chronic inflammation and scarring.

2.1.5 Insulin-like growth factor (IGF)

Insulin-like Growth Factors (IGFs) are primarily synthesized in the liver, but their role in wound healing gains particular interest due to their secondary production by fibroblasts and their release from platelets during clotting. These growth factors are crucial for stimulating keratinocyte and fibroblast mitogenesis, promoting cellular activity, and driving cellular differentiation.

Insulin-like Growth Factor-1 (IGF-1), also known as somatomedin-C, has garnered significant attention in wound healing research from various perspectives. It plays a pivotal role in the migration of both keratinocytes and fibroblasts and can upregulate the expression of hyaluronan synthase genes, thereby influencing the synthesis of hyaluronic acid, a key extracellular matrix component in wound repair. More recent mechanistic studies in a rat model of wound healing have demonstrated that IGF-1 can effectively reduce inflammation, enhance vascular regeneration, improve re-epithelialization, and promote collagen deposition in acute wounds [53]. These findings underscore its potential for further therapeutic development in wound care.

A recombinant form of IGF-1 (rhIGF-1) is already approved for treating certain human conditions, such as IGF-1 deficiency, and for neural protection. Furthermore, ongoing medical applications are actively exploring the development of new medications based on rhIGF-1 for a broader range of diseases, including its promising use in tissue regeneration and wound healing.

2.1.6 Collagen metabolism/deposition factors and inhibitors

Parallel to direct growth factor interventions, other clinical development strategies for scar management have focused on targeting different pathways involved in collagen deposition. Early clinical trials utilizing collagen cross-linking agents are noteworthy in this context. One such agent, beta-aminopropionitrile (BAPN), a lysyl oxidase (LOX) inhibitor that acts by chelating a required copper ion cofactor, was investigated for its potential to ameliorate scar formation. However, BAPN encountered issues with toxicity or hypersensitivity, leading to its discontinuation in further investigations for several decades. Nevertheless, renewed interest has emerged recently following the development of new topical formulations.

Indeed, a topically applied, designed pan-lysyl oxidase inhibitor, PXS-6302, has shown promising results, leading to improved scar appearance without overt scarring in porcine models and demonstrating preliminary positive effects in human scar management. Consequently, an Australian group is currently investigating this compound for its potential in other fibrotic diseases [54]. In contrast, another copper-chelating agent, D-penicillamine, has been used in the management of fibrosis in scleroderma patients, with some clinical groups advocating for its benefit in this rheumatologic cohort [55]. This drug exerts several effects on collagen metabolism, notably an inhibition of collagen biosynthesis, which demonstrates beneficial anti-fibrotic properties and leads to reduced skin thickening with continued use in patients afflicted by this debilitating disease. Further research to elucidate the mechanisms of action in these severely affected patients could provide critical insights for the development of broad anti-fibrotic treatments and enhanced scar management strategies.

Beyond collagen cross-linking, other growth factors and inhibitors are under clinical investigation due to their implication in fibrosis. Prominent among these is Connective Tissue Growth Factor (CTGF), a key mediator involved in cell proliferation and differentiation, making it a compelling therapeutic target. Several clinical trials are currently in Phase II using siRNA preparations targeting CTGF for skin scarring, specifically with inhibitors named OLX-10010 and RXI-109. The latter, following an announcement of positive patient reactivity by the company (then RXi Pharmaceuticals), saw its parent company rebrand to Phio Pharmaceuticals Corp. in 2018, shifting its focus toward next-generation immuno-oncology therapeutics, and subsequently, further development for scar management appeared to cease. More recently, in 2023, the CTGF inhibitor OLX10010, developed by OliX Pharmaceuticals Inc., announced significant improvement in hypertrophic scar appearance in its Phase II clinical trials following intradermal administration compared to placebo. However, safety data from this trial have not yet been announced in parallel. To date, there is no peer-reviewed clinical publication detailing these specific findings, though they are listed in several clinical trial databases [56].

Overall, attempting to devise single-molecule development strategies for achieving scarless wound healing may be overly optimistic, as attested by several decades of both preclinical and clinical work. A more promising approach involves assessing the intricate pathways leading to scarless wound healing at the fetal level and drawing comparisons with the fibrotic pathways observed in adult disease. Distinguishing the key elements between these two extremes could provide common ground for understanding critical mechanisms. Research can then target multiple individual molecules to improve scarring in adult wounds, aiming to emulate the regenerative outcomes seen in fetal wound healing.

However, a complementary and perhaps more impactful avenue may lie in remaining at the whole-cell level with cell therapies. This approach concentrates on standardized cell sources and manufacturing processes, coupled with innovative patient-oriented treatment plans tailored to specific wound types, sizes, and inflammatory statuses.

3. Biological strategies of scarless wound healing

Before the advent of advanced cell cultures for patient graft development, various cutaneous preparations, both animal and human, were crucial for managing severe burns and wounds by containing fluid loss and mitigating infection. Cadaveric skin from human and porcine sources was routinely employed. Over time, this evolved into a diverse array of acellular and cellular tissue constructs designed for skin regeneration and scar management.

Historically, as early as 1949, the US Navy Skin Bank in Bethesda, Maryland, pioneered human skin banking for extensive total body surface burns. Their rigorous screening protocols for contaminants revealed that only 54 out of over 1112 cadaveric donors were deemed unsuitable, primarily due to bacterial and fungal contamination [57]. In the 1960s, the French Navy utilized fetal bovine dermis, a material rich in Type III collagen, for burn treatments (personal communication, Prof. Louis Rey). It took many decades for a similar product to gain FDA approval: PriMatrix (TEI Biosciences Inc., Boston, Massachusetts), a dermal substitute derived from fetal bovine skin, which proved effective in supporting split-thickness skin grafting, initially demonstrated in complicated hand burns [58]. This company was subsequently acquired by Integra LifeSciences (Princeton, NJ, USA) in 2015 for a cash closing of $312 million.

The late 1990s brought significant concerns regarding patient safety, particularly in Europe, due to the potential transmission of prions associated with bovine and human-derived products (e.g., cadaveric skin) entering the medical device market. This crisis directly impacted clinical practice; for instance, our Swiss Burn Center experienced a rupture in its supply of human cadaver skin from the Euroskin Bank for severe burn patients, necessitating the urgent identification of alternative solutions. During this critical period, frozen and glycerol-preserved porcine skin emerged as a vital "first cover" for severe burn patients within our National Burn Center.

The decades that followed witnessed a rapid evolution in skin grafting substitutes and dermal matrices available on the market, which have been comprehensively reviewed in recent years [59]. Many biological matrices have emerged, serving not only as temporary covers for burns and wounds but also facilitating one- or two-stage surgical repairs (e.g., preparing the dermal structure for a secondary skin graft). These diverse products originate from various sources:

1. Porcine: Examples include Biobrane™, a nylon membrane coated with porcine collagen type I.

2. Bovine collagen: Integra® is a bilayer construct of cross-linked bovine collagen with chondroitin-6-sulfate on a silicone membrane.

3. Human cadaveric transformed dermis: Alloderm® consists of lyophilized, de-epithelialized dermis.

4. Bacterial fermentation of hyaluronic acid: Hyalomatrix® is HA associated with a semi-permeable silicone membrane.

5. Porcine intestine: Oasis® Wound Matrix is an acellular small intestine mucosa.

6. Fetal bovine skin: PriMatrix® is a fetal bovine skin derivative.

Numerous other similar formulations and components have been reported in the aforementioned reviews [59, 60]. More recently, different fish skin preparations have also gained traction for burn coverage and treatment. Notable examples include Kerecis™, an acellular fish skin derived from Atlantic cod [61], and tilapia skin, which has been explored for patient care in Brazil and India [62].

Many of these biological substrates have also provided crucial support for the subsequent advancements in cellular therapy and cell delivery systems for wound and burn management. A significant number have been effectively used in conjunction with conventional skin grafting to help prepare a more robust dermal structure and enhance overall skin repair outcomes [63].

3.1 Central importance of cellular therapies in burns and wounds

While autologous skin grafts remain the gold standard for treating extensive skin loss, their application presents significant challenges in cases of extensive burns where donor skin may be insufficient or when the wound bed is heavily contaminated. To overcome these limitations, cellular therapies for wound healing have emerged, showcasing a remarkable evolution in cell types, origins, and formulations (**Figure 2**, right column).

Many early therapies, particularly those developed for burn patients, originated from patient biopsies, utilizing both keratinocyte and fibroblast cultures in cell therapy and tissue engineering products. These approaches often involved *ex vivo* cell culture expansion to ensure sufficient quantities for patient treatment, especially when large surface areas required coverage. For decades, several preparations using autologous cells (derived from the patient themselves) have been established, including Cultured Epidermal Autografts (CEAs), which comprise patient-derived keratinocytes alone, and Cultured Dermal/Epidermal Autografts (CDEAs), which incorporate both patient keratinocytes and fibroblasts. A major hurdle with these methods has been the time required to generate sufficient cells for timely patient treatment.

CEAs and CDEAs have been integrated into routine patient care in institutions possessing appropriate accredited cell culture facilities and trained personnel. CEA production typically necessitates 2–3 weeks, while the inclusion of fibroblasts in CDEA extends the manufacturing process to approximately 6 weeks. Although these autologous approaches offer distinct advantages over split-thickness skin grafts, they are characterized by lengthy production times, inherent fragility, and high costs, particularly outside specialized hospital settings equipped with good manufacturing practices (GMP) manufacturing capabilities. The critical challenge remains the turnaround time for generating adequate cell numbers. Current clinical practice generally reserves CDEA use for patients with burns exceeding 70% total body surface area (TBSA), allowing sufficient time for the production of autologous skin fibroblasts. A significant advantage of combining keratinocytes and fibroblasts in CDEA is the notably improved final skin reconstruction outcome, including reduced tissue contraction. This benefit is particularly valuable for challenging anatomical sites, such as joints and the neck/face region, where minimizing skin contracture is paramount. However, crucial considerations include the source and manufacturing methods of fibroblasts, as their characteristics can vary significantly depending on the harvest site, tissue origin, age, and processing techniques [64, 65].

Acknowledging the significant manufacturing delays associated with CEA and CDEA, recent advancements have focused on enabling more rapid growth of patient keratinocytes without the need for feeder layers, effectively reducing the time to cell availability to approximately 10–12 days [66]. Furthermore, exploring the potential cellular differences between adult and fetal fibroblasts offers profound insights into the mechanisms underpinning scar-free tissue regeneration, a phenomenon consistently documented both *in vitro* and *in vivo* in human and animal models [3, 5–8, 67–69].

More recently, other diverse cell sources have been, and continue to be, investigated in clinical trials worldwide as potential candidates for generating larger cell stocks for more rapid treatment paradigms. These include stem cells derived from bone marrow (BM-MSC), adipose tissue (AD-MSC or ASC), umbilical cord (UM-MSC), placenta, peripheral blood, hair follicles, keratinocyte progenitors, dental pulp (DPSC), and excised burn skin (BD-MSC), as comprehensively reviewed by Rangatchew et al. concerning inflammation and wound healing of thermal skin burns [70]. These cells can be derived from autogenic, allogeneic, or xenogeneic origins and from various developmental ages. Numerous advancements in cell therapies for burn and wound management have yielded significant observations, including rapid wound healing, skin regeneration with soft tissue augmentation, increased collagen deposition, inhibition of scar tissue formation, effects on pain management, reduction of inflammatory responses, and even systemic effects related to metabolism, inflammation, and immunosuppression.

However, the widespread expansion of cell therapies for routine clinical use has primarily been hindered by factors related to the cell sources themselves, such as their differentiation capacity, potential for cell fusion, and the need for appropriate mechanisms that ensure effective growth factor crosstalk with biomaterials and delivery systems following transplantation. In response to these challenges, new formulations described as "cell-free therapies" have emerged globally. These involve products like exosomes, secretomes, extracellular vesicles, cellular lysates, or conditioned media. While conceptually "cell-free" in their final application, it is crucial to recognize that from a manufacturing perspective, they are indeed more complex, as their "raw starting materials" are live cell sources, necessitating varying degrees of intricate processing for purification. Importantly, cell therapies are gaining increased clinical acceptance, primarily because whole cells intrinsically contain a comprehensive array of growth factors, cytokines, and proteins, which are released in a sustained manner, optimally corresponding to the needs of local stimuli that influence positive wound healing within the local microenvironment. Given that all cell sources contain specific secretomes and by-products such as exosomes and conditioned media with such contained factors, further preclinical and clinical research must center on rigorously evaluating whether these highly manipulated subfractions are as efficient as the whole cells themselves.

Burn injuries represent a significant global health challenge, affecting over 11 million individuals annually. These injuries impose a profound impact, leading to high morbidity and mortality rates, as well as enduring psychological and economic consequences [71, 72]. Historically, up to 90% of burn injuries occurred in low- and middle-income countries, with children and the elderly disproportionately affected. However, the recent increase in global conflicts may significantly alter this trend. Therefore, the development of effective and readily available cell-based therapies for burn wound and scar management is critically important, particularly for managing patient populations in diverse and resource-limited environments [73, 74]. Indeed, cell therapies offer significant promise, surpassing conventional approaches in their ability to stimulate comprehensive tissue regeneration. These therapies have consistently demonstrated remarkable efficacy in promoting angiogenesis, epithelialization, granulation tissue formation, and collagen deposition, and possess potent anti-oxidative and anti-inflammatory properties that inhibit apoptosis [75–81]. For nearly four decades, cellular therapies have been a cornerstone in the treatment of severe burns, primarily with the goal of saving lives. The ongoing evolution of cell types and formulations has enabled the optimization of treatments across the different phases of wound healing.

Burn injuries are inherently dynamic and can progress in severity over time, characterized by prolonged inflammation, impaired blood flow to the affected area, and ultimately, tissue necrosis [76, 77]. The intermediate stage of a burn injury, often referred to as the stasis zone, may offer a critical window for therapeutic intervention. Timely and effective treatments during this period are crucial to prevent the progression of the burn depth and promote optimal wound healing. The overarching clinical goal is to develop novel interventions that effectively minimize inflammation, stimulate the regenerative process, and ultimately minimize scarring [82].

3.2 Key complementary contributions of fibroblasts and keratinocytes in burn wound healing

It has been well-established that combining keratinocytes with fibroblasts leads to improved clinical outcomes for burn patients [76, 83]. Several mechanisms contribute to this enhanced efficacy, as evidenced by both developmental and clinical research. Historically, it was challenging to culture keratinocytes in the laboratory without the support of fibroblasts or fibroblast feeder layers. While patient fibroblasts could be used, they often overgrew the keratinocyte cultures. To address this, early clinical trials employed irradiated 3 T3 mouse embryo cells as a feeder layer, following the protocols established by Rheinwald and Green [84]. While xeno-free media systems have been explored for laboratory research, their translation to clinical use has been limited to date. Many media formulations are not able to adequately support keratinocyte stratification, which was desired for CEA and CDEA preparations. Therefore, alternative formulation approaches (e.g., cell sprays) have been developed to enable earlier patient treatment with cell therapies, even without fully stratified cell sheets [80, 81, 85, 86].

Important advancements allowing significant time reduction for cultured keratinocytes for severe burn patients are primordial for enabling earlier initiation of patient therapies. Development of clinical-grade media designed specifically for keratinocyte growth also has to be manufactured with advanced certification, such as those offered by CELLnTEC (Higher Certified [HC], Bern, Switzerland), as this progress is mandatory for regulatory requirements to support clinical trials.

3.3 Outlook on the commercial applications of cutaneous cell therapy protocols and products

Past clinical experience with keratinocyte- and fibroblast-based cell therapies has yielded invaluable insights, particularly regarding the influence of cell source age (adult vs. neonatal), the ratios of different cell types within a formulation, and their efficacy across various clinical applications (e.g., severe burns versus chronic ulcers). While initial interest predominantly focused on burn wound treatment, the market for chronic wound therapies has become increasingly prominent. This shift is partly attributable to a global decline in severe burn incidence and the substantial logistical challenges associated with mass-producing cell-based products for the extensive surface areas frequently affected by burns. Consequently, researchers have actively explored alternative, readily available sources of fibroblasts and keratinocytes.

Fibroblasts and keratinocytes derived from newborn foreskin have been extensively utilized in wound healing research and for the development of advanced skin graft substrates. A prominent example is Apligraf® (Organogenesis, Canton, MA, USA), which received FDA approval in 1998 for the treatment of venous ulcers and subsequently for diabetic foot ulcers in 2000. This innovative product incorporates a combination of fibroblasts and keratinocytes cultured on a bovine collagen matrix, forming a stratified, living skin substitute. Apligraf® has also been adapted for oral mucosal applications under the brand name Gintuit® (Organogenesis). This approval was specifically for topical application to surgically created vascularized wounds in mucogingival conditions, utilizing the same formulation as the wound care product. This successful adaptation highlights the significant potential for repurposing existing cell-based therapies for diverse clinical indications.

In 2009, Goedkoop et al. conducted a pivotal study utilizing growth-arrested keratinocytes and fibroblasts derived from adult discarded tissues obtained during breast reconstruction surgery [65]. These cells were combined within a fibrinogen-thrombin matrix and delivered *via* a spray method. This approach facilitated the initial investigation of growth factors relevant to wound healing in a Phase I clinical trial, enabling the evaluation of different cell ratios (i.e., keratinocytes to fibroblasts) and doses [65].

The initial Phase I safety study involved 14 patients with chronic venous leg ulcers unresponsive to standard treatments. Weekly applications of the growth-arrested cells were administered for 12 consecutive weeks, evaluating various cell ratios (1:9 and 1:1 keratinocytes to fibroblasts) and doses (2.5, 5.0, and 10×10^6 cells/mL). Overall, the Phase I study identified a keratinocyte-to-fibroblast ratio of 1:9 and a dose of 5×10^6 cells/mL as the most promising combination for further investigation in a Phase II clinical trial [87].

The product known as HP802-247, also referred to as Allox, underwent a complex development journey. Initially manufactured by Modex Thérapeutiques SA (Lausanne, Switzerland), it was later acquired by Isotis SA (Lausanne, Switzerland), and subsequently by DFB Pharmaceuticals (Fort Worth, TX, USA), which was then acquired by Healthpoint Biotherapeutics (Fort Worth, TX, USA). Notably, the cell source for this product shifted from adult skin biopsies (obtained during breast reconstruction) to newborn foreskin cells for the Phase II clinical trial [65, 87]. The Phase II study evaluated different dosing regimens, applying cell doses of 0.5×10^6 and 5×10^6 cells at intervals of 7 and 14 days for a total of 12 weeks. Interestingly, the lower dose (0.5×10^6 cells) administered at the longer interval (14 days) demonstrated the most effective results [87].

Following the successful completion of the Phase II trial, Smith & Nephew (London, UK) acquired the product. More recently, Healiva (Lugano, Switzerland; part of the Bioseutica Group, Lugano, Switzerland) announced the acquisition of this technology, signaling a renewed focus on the original Epidex technology developed by Modex for autologous skin substitutes. In addition to this acquisition, Healiva announced the purchase of allogeneic fibroblast cells from B. Braun (Melsungen, Germany) [88]. This strategic move aims to enhance the cell culture potential of patient-derived outer root sheath keratinocytes by combining them with a readily available allogeneic fibroblast cell source. A key advantage of this approach is the elimination of the need for a surgical procedure to obtain autologous skin for the development of the skin substitute, as keratinocytes can be readily obtained from plucked hair follicles of the patients. While promising, this approach would still require a substantial amount of time for culturing outer root sheath keratinocytes, potentially creating a bottleneck in rapid patient treatment. However, focusing initially on smaller chronic wounds appears more practical for scaling up keratinocyte production. Healiva has announced plans to further develop allogeneic formulations, although the specific cell types have not yet been disclosed, with availability projected for 2027.

Interestingly, in 2015, the Korean company Tego Science (Seoul, Korea) introduced a line of skin replacement and repair products under the brand name KeraHeal®. KeraHeal-Allo®, an allogeneic, off-the-shelf product within this line, utilizes newborn foreskin fibroblasts and keratinocytes delivered in a convenient spray format. KeraHeal-Allo® underwent clinical trials evaluating three different cell doses: a low concentration (6.7×10^6 cells/1.5 mL), a medium concentration (20×10^6 cells/1.5 mL), and a high concentration (60×10^6 cells/1.5 mL) [89]. Clinical studies demonstrated that the medium concentration exhibited the most rapid wound healing while maintaining safety for deep second-degree burns. This medium concentration was subsequently selected for Phase III trials and ultimately approved for clinical use [90]. The hydrogel-based delivery system of KeraHeal-Allo® offers a significant advantage for treating large surface area burns due to its ease of application.

Finally, several medical devices have been developed to facilitate the processing of small patient skin biopsies directly at the point of care. These devices enable the rapid preparation of cell sprays for direct local application after being processed using specific methods. Examples include ReCell™ (Avita Medical [Valencia, CA, USA], approved in California and Australia at the end of 2023), CellMist™ and SkinGun™ (RenovaCare [Scottsdale, AZ, USA]), and Viticell™ (IBSA, France and Switzerland). These devices have significantly improved patient accessibility and can enzymatically digest all relevant cell populations, including keratinocytes, fibroblasts, and melanocytes, to create a ready-to-use cell spray for application to larger surface areas [91]. However, it is important to note that without *ex vivo* cell expansion, these devices are not suitable for treating patients with severe burns covering extensive body surface areas. They are more appropriate for smaller wounds and burns, particularly when used in conjunction with large meshed skin grafts. A key limitation for widespread adoption remains the substantial cost of these medical device kits, often several thousand dollars.

It is worth mentioning that as early as the 1990s, clinical use of frozen allogeneic human epidermal cultured sheets (derived from a human epidermal cell strain, HE-120, obtained from the foreskin of a newborn donor from a low-risk HIV population, with cells at passage 4 being HIV tested) was routinely practiced in Mexico for complicated leg ulcers. This method provided ready-to-use frozen preparations for patient application with high success rates [92].

3.4 Progenitor cell therapy and off-the-shelf formulations

The diverse cell populations currently employed in clinical settings for burn and wound management often possess stem cell characteristics, particularly their differentiation potential. While this multipotency offers an advantage for various medical applications, it also presents a challenge: maintaining a specific cell phenotype in culture may not be fully guaranteed once the cells are introduced into a patient, as the complex *in vivo* microenvironment contains numerous growth factors and cytokines that can influence cellular fate. Therefore, establishing a stable cell source that is not prone to unwanted differentiation upon implantation is highly desirable.

Dermal fibroblast progenitors exhibit remarkable homogeneity and stability. Their origin from a defined developmental stage, coupled with their unimodal cultured cell populations, inherent absence of differentiation potential, and high resistance to oxidative stress and cryopreservation, makes them a compelling candidate [24, 93, 94]. Histological analysis of tissues used to initiate these cell cultures further supports that the uniform quality of the resulting cell cultures may be attributed to the lack of specific "niches" or microenvironments that might otherwise promote heterogeneity in cells derived from younger or older aged tissues.

For robust cell expansion and cell banking potential in burn and wound management, allogeneic progenitor fibroblasts (FE002-SK2) have been utilized for several decades. Historically, these cells have primarily been employed in clinical trials and have not yet been developed as a final commercial living cell product. A significant advantage of this cell source, which is typically derived from a single organ donation, is its immediate accessibility for patient use. This is because extensive master and working cell banks can be established under cGMP (current Good Manufacturing Practices) conditions, making them readily available for clinical trial authorization and rapid deployment.

To date, progenitor cells offer a safe and consistent cell source for early treatment protocols requiring tegument cover. In Lausanne, Switzerland, our team has implemented the use of progenitor fibroblasts (PFF) in clinical care for over

15 years. We have demonstrated that these cells can be incorporated into early treatment, as early as 4–5 days postburn, by providing a crucial first cover for the patient, akin to temporary covers like cadaveric or porcine skin [82, 95]. Furthermore, PFF can be strategically utilized to create a robust dermal substrate, facilitating the subsequent delivery of patient keratinocytes to form a Cultured Dermal/Epidermal Autograft (CDEA) with two cell types. This approach effectively circumvents the complexities and delays associated with co-culturing and delivering both fibroblasts and keratinocytes simultaneously. Because PFF can be prepared and cryopreserved in advance, they can be combined with patient-derived keratinocytes as soon as these latter cells are available and tested for efficient attachment to dermal tissue substrates (DED). Instead of enduring the 40–60 days typically required for traditional combined cell therapy protocols, a new paradigm can be established, leveraging readily available cell sources to optimize the maximum surface area for debridement in severe burn patients (50–90% TBSA). Critically, these PFF cell stocks can be prepared on the day of surgical intervention, enabling optimal and timely patient care.

Progenitor fibroblasts distinguish themselves by providing all the necessary factors to support scarless wound healing across various types of lesions, including burns, pressure ulcers, and chronic wounds. These cells actively secrete a regenerative extracellular matrix (ECM) that is notably enriched in Type III collagen, fibronectin, and hyaluronic acid. This unique ECM composition collectively promotes keratinocyte migration, enhances re-epithelialization, and facilitates proper dermal remodeling. The predominance of Type III collagen, which is characteristic of fetal and early wound healing environments, is associated with a more organized and less fibrotic matrix deposition, a stark contrast to the Type I collagen that dominates in adult fibroblasts and is strongly linked to scar formation and fibrosis [96].

Moreover, fetal progenitor fibroblasts exhibit a unique cytokine expression profile, notably characterized by high levels of Transforming Growth Factor-beta 3 (TGF-β3). TGF-β3 plays a pivotal role in modulating wound healing by actively suppressing pro-fibrotic signaling pathways and promoting regeneration over fibrotic repair. In stark contrast, adult fibroblasts demonstrate sustained expression of TGF-β1 and TGF-β2. These isoforms activate the Smad 2 and 3 signaling pathway, vigorously stimulate Type I collagen production, and drive the differentiation of fibroblasts into myofibroblasts, thereby contributing decisively to scar formation. Importantly, progenitor fibroblasts show limited and transient expression of alpha-smooth muscle actin (α-SMA), which signifies a reduction in their conversion into contractile myofibroblasts. This diminished myofibroblast activity is directly associated with reduced wound contraction and a lower risk of hypertrophic scarring [96].

While adult dermal fibroblasts undoubtedly play a crucial role in skin repair, their fibrotic potential is well-documented and tends to increase with the patient's age. These cells are inherently heterogeneous and exhibit significant variability in their differentiation capacity from patient to patient, leading to unpredictable biological responses. This inherent variability poses a major challenge for tissue-engineering strategies that frequently rely on autologous fibroblasts. Furthermore, the substantial time required for their isolation, culture, and expansion, especially when combined with autologous keratinocytes, can significantly delay the initiation of treatment, severely limiting their applicability in clinical settings that demand rapid therapeutic interventions.

The inherent heterogeneity of fibroblast populations within burn wounds underscores the critical importance of carefully selecting the appropriate cell source for optimal outcomes. Varkey et al. already demonstrated in 2014 the significance of fibroblast origin by comparing superficial dermal fibroblasts to those derived from deeper layers of the dermis (**Figure 3**) [68]. Their study, utilizing a tissue-engineered skin model, revealed that superficial dermal fibroblasts, when combined with keratinocytes, exhibited enhanced dermo-epidermal adhesion and anchoring protein expression, resulting in the formation of a continuous epidermis with improved barrier function. Furthermore, these superficial fibroblast-keratinocyte combinations demonstrated higher expression levels of epidermal proteins, such as keratin-5 and E-cadherin, and exhibited more robust basement membranes with increased levels of laminin-5, nidogen, and type VII collagen, compared to combinations using deep dermal fibroblasts [68].

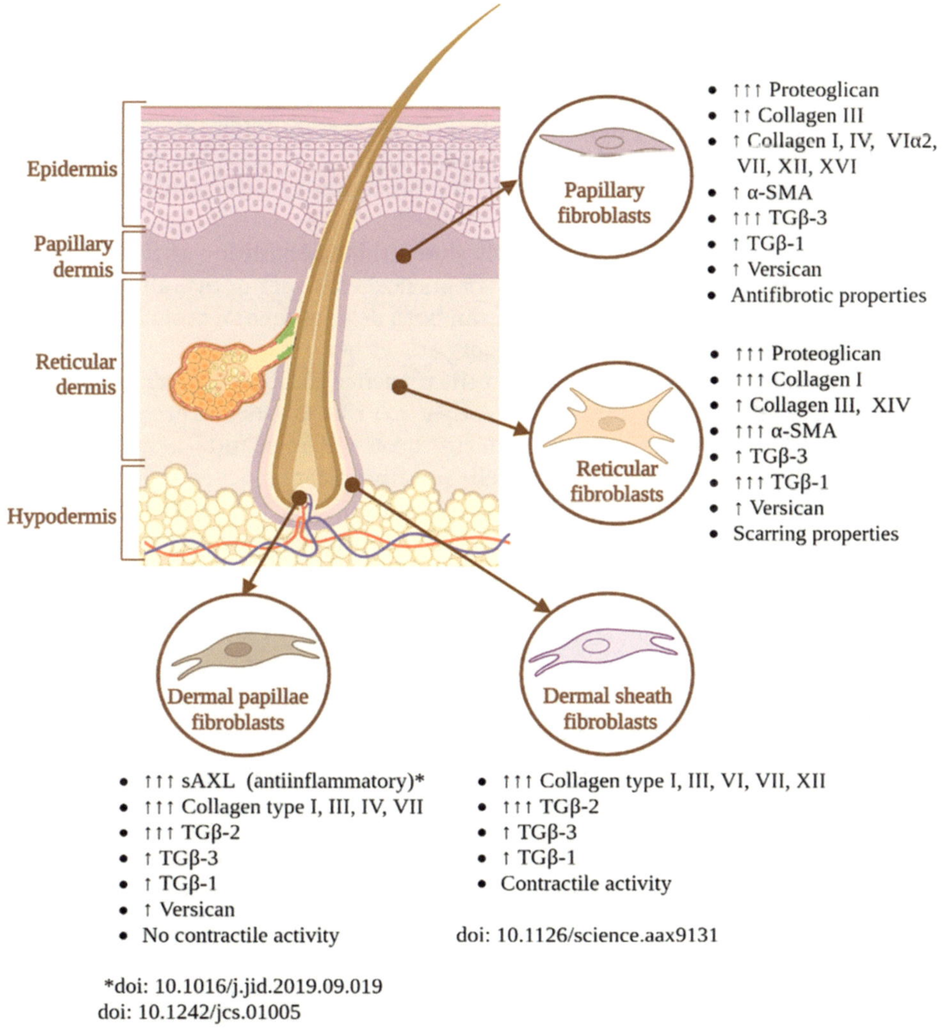

Figure 3.
Fibroblast niches within the skin localization. Fibroblasts are derived from papillary dermis, reticular dermis, and two other sources within the hypodermis. Each specific fibroblast origin specifies different mechanistic actions (quantity represented by a scale of ↑ to ↑↑↑) related to wound healing and scar formation.

4. Discussion

The escalating incidence of severe burns and complex wounds, including those resulting from increasing international conflicts and radiation exposure, necessitates the development of highly effective and targeted cellular and tissue therapies. The inherent potency of cell therapies offers a significant advantage over conventional therapeutic approaches. These advanced modalities have consistently demonstrated efficient tissue regenerative processes, encompassing enhanced angiogenesis, robust epithelialization, rapid granulation tissue formation, optimal soft tissue development, and organized collagen deposition. Moreover, cellular therapies exhibit potent anti-oxidative and anti-inflammatory properties that effectively inhibit apoptosis, a critical factor in mitigating tissue damage.

Burn injuries are dynamic, often progressing in severity and depth over time, leading to prolonged, excessive inflammation, impaired tissue perfusion, and ultimately, widespread apoptosis and tissue necrosis. The intermediate stage of burn injury, known as the zone of stasis, represents a potentially salvageable area. Therefore, timely and effective interventions during this critical window are paramount for preventing burn progression and initiating comprehensive wound healing. The overarching goal is to develop novel interventions that eliminate or significantly attenuate inflammation, stimulate the healing process, and ultimately achieve minimal scarring.

Clinical experience to date consistently shows that the addition of fibroblasts to keratinocytes in the treatment of burn patients leads to superior overall outcomes [76, 83]. Several mechanisms, deduced from both developmental biology and clinical observations, likely contribute to this synergistic effect. Historically, it was challenging to grow keratinocytes *in vitro* without the presence of fibroblasts or fibroblast feeder layers. To circumvent the problem of patient fibroblasts overgrowing keratinocytes, early clinical trials, following the protocols of Green and Rheinwald, incorporated irradiated mouse 3 T3 embryo cells as a fibroblast feeder source. While other groups have successfully utilized patient-derived feeder layers or alternative cell types [97], significant efforts have also focused on developing feeder-free media systems with defined or animal-origin-free components for laboratory research. However, few of these media formulations have progressed to clinical acceptance [98]. Many early media developments overlooked that keratinocytes grown in serum-free conditions might not stratify effectively. Nevertheless, alternatives to fully stratified culture sheets, such as cell sprays, have emerged for patient burn care, enabling earlier treatment initiation. More recently, human keratinocytes and other skin cell populations, including fibroblasts and melanocytes, can be efficiently cultured and prepared for clinical use without feeder layers, utilizing defined growth media [66]. This advancement now allows for the efficient growth of keratinocytes directly from patient biopsies within approximately 10 days, providing sufficient cell sources to begin earlier patient therapy [66, 67]. Furthermore, clinical-grade media are continuously being improved for keratinocyte growth, such as those from CELLnTEC (Higher Certified (HC), Bern, Switzerland), which are suitable for Phase I and II clinical trials.

The enhanced efficacy observed when fibroblasts and keratinocytes are combined in cell therapy regimens suggests that extracellular matrix (ECM) synthesis and soluble factors are crucial for the successful development of keratinocyte grafts for patients. These two major cell types actively respond to the inflammatory phase in cutaneous repair and regeneration after burns and wounds. Their continuous communication and paracrine crosstalk are essential for achieving normal tissue restoration. Consequently, the early use of fibroblasts in burn therapy can effectively prepare proper granulation tissue and wound bed, ensuring efficient attachment and integration of keratinocytes.

The inherent heterogeneity of fibroblasts from burn patients and the judicious selection of the appropriate cell population are paramount for optimizing the formation of the dermo-epidermal interface. Varkey et al. highlighted this by comparing superficial dermal fibroblasts to those derived from deeper dermal layers. Their study, using a tissue-engineered skin model (collagen-glycosaminoglycan matrix), revealed that superficial dermal fibroblasts, when combined with keratinocytes, exhibited enhanced dermo-epidermal adhesion and anchoring protein expression, leading to the formation of a continuous epidermis with improved barrier function. Moreover, superficial fibroblast-keratinocyte combinations demonstrated higher expression levels of epidermal proteins like keratin-5 and E-cadherin and showed more robust basement membranes with increased levels of laminin-5, nidogen, and type VII collagen, compared to combinations utilizing deep dermal fibroblasts [68].

Currently available tissue-engineering strategies often employ heterogeneous populations of dermal fibroblasts, which exhibit variability in differentiation capacity among patient donors (**Figure 3**). Regardless, the use of autologous patient fibroblasts for immediate treatment remains challenging due to the protracted time required for culturing sufficient cells for combination with patient keratinocytes. Furthermore, it is well-established that adult fibroblasts contribute to fibrotic characteristics in wound healing, a physiological capacity that changes with developmental age.

Historically, the utilization of cell sources has evolved from a primary focus on "saving lives" in severe burns to encompassing chronic wound care for recalcitrant ulcers and rapidly repairing open wounds in general. The ultimate healed skin outcome and the drive to achieve perfect skin repair are intimately linked to the choice of "effector" cells used in cell therapy development. We have gained significant insights from developmental medicine in this regard. It is well-documented that dermal fibroblasts from early gestation exhibit dramatically different wound healing patterns compared to those from late gestation or adult stages. These profound differences in tissues and cells contribute to the presence or absence of scarring during skin regeneration and repair.

The major factor previously identified as being related to scarless wound healing was the pattern of collagen deposition derived from fibroblasts, leading to the hypothesis that fibroblasts within wounds are the "major effector cells" controlling wound healing outcomes [69]. Fetal fibroblasts are central to the overall process of wound repair by creating an optimal microenvironment that fosters lower inflammation and allows for the organized interstitial structure of tissue. The production, deposition, and remodeling of the ECM by fibroblasts crucially distinguish scarless tissue remodeling based on the nature and pattern of the matrix deposition [99]. Therefore, the mammalian fetus demonstrably exhibits processes of true regeneration, characterized by the restoration of tissue to its normal skin architecture without inflammation, without the associated contraction of surrounding tissue, and without the formation of a scar.

The fundamental differences between fetal and postnatal wound healing have been extensively studied at both the molecular and protein expression levels. While numerous individual proteins have been identified in the pathway for scarless wound healing, most therapeutic developments to date have unfortunately not yielded major progress in this domain.

Overall, devising single-molecule development strategies for scarless wound healing may prove to be overly optimistic, as evidenced by several decades of preclinical and clinical work. A more productive approach involves meticulously assessing the pathways that lead to scarless wound healing at the fetal level and drawing direct comparisons with the fibrotic pathways observed in adult disease. Distinguishing the key elements between these two extremes may provide common ground for understanding critical mechanisms. Research can then strategically target multiple individual molecules to improve scarring seen in adult wounds, striving to emulate the regenerative outcomes observed in fetal wound healing. However, it may also be highly beneficial to focus on whole-cell therapies, concentrating on standardized cell sources and manufacturing processes, coupled with innovative, patient-oriented treatment plans tailored to the specific wound type, size, and inflammatory status.

5. Conclusions and future prospects

The global scar treatment market is projected to reach an estimated value of 50–60 billion USD by 2030. This significant growth is driven by several factors, including the increasing prevalence of skin diseases, a persistent incidence of burn injuries, the expanding field of aesthetic surgery, and continuous advancements in biotechnology and scar management strategies.

A wide range of skin conditions, such as hypertrophic scars, constrictive scars, keloids, burns, acne scars, postsurgical scars, and stretch marks, are currently addressed through both invasive and noninvasive treatments. Among these, laser technology plays a crucial role by facilitating cellular reorganization within existing scars, promoting the proper orientation and construction of the extracellular matrix (ECM) for more sustainable tissue repair.

Despite advancements, a high percentage of burn injuries continue to result in unacceptable scarring. Even today, skin grafting remains the gold standard for treating second- and third-degree burns. However, it is increasingly supplemented by tissue-engineered skin substitutes and parallel therapies. These complementary approaches are designed not only to expedite wound healing but also to ensure improved aesthetic outcomes and comprehensive scar management.

Mechanisms related to growth factors (GFs), various cellular components, and novel cell therapies are steadily advancing, becoming central to innovative approaches for modulating the intricate pathway of wound healing and scar management. As wound management, particularly for burn patients, has evolved significantly beyond mere survival, there is a distinct and growing focus on optimizing the quality of regenerated skin.

Much emphasis has been given to slow-release formulations and also to combined growth factor delivery [12]. For biologicals, slow-release formulations using hydrogels may be a good solution not only for delivery but also for stabilization (**Figure 4**).

At least for biological formulations, unraveling the most pertinent cell sources and their precise roles may be the key to achieving the ultimate paradigm of perfect skin regeneration, as a combination of many growth factors/cytokines is involved in the intricate pathway [100].

Regulatory framework complexity may present major obstacles for cell therapy implementation in the clinic. Even though over the last two decades there has been a positive evolution, it is imperative to continue improvements in regulation to ensure safe, effective, and high-quality biological therapeutic development for patients.

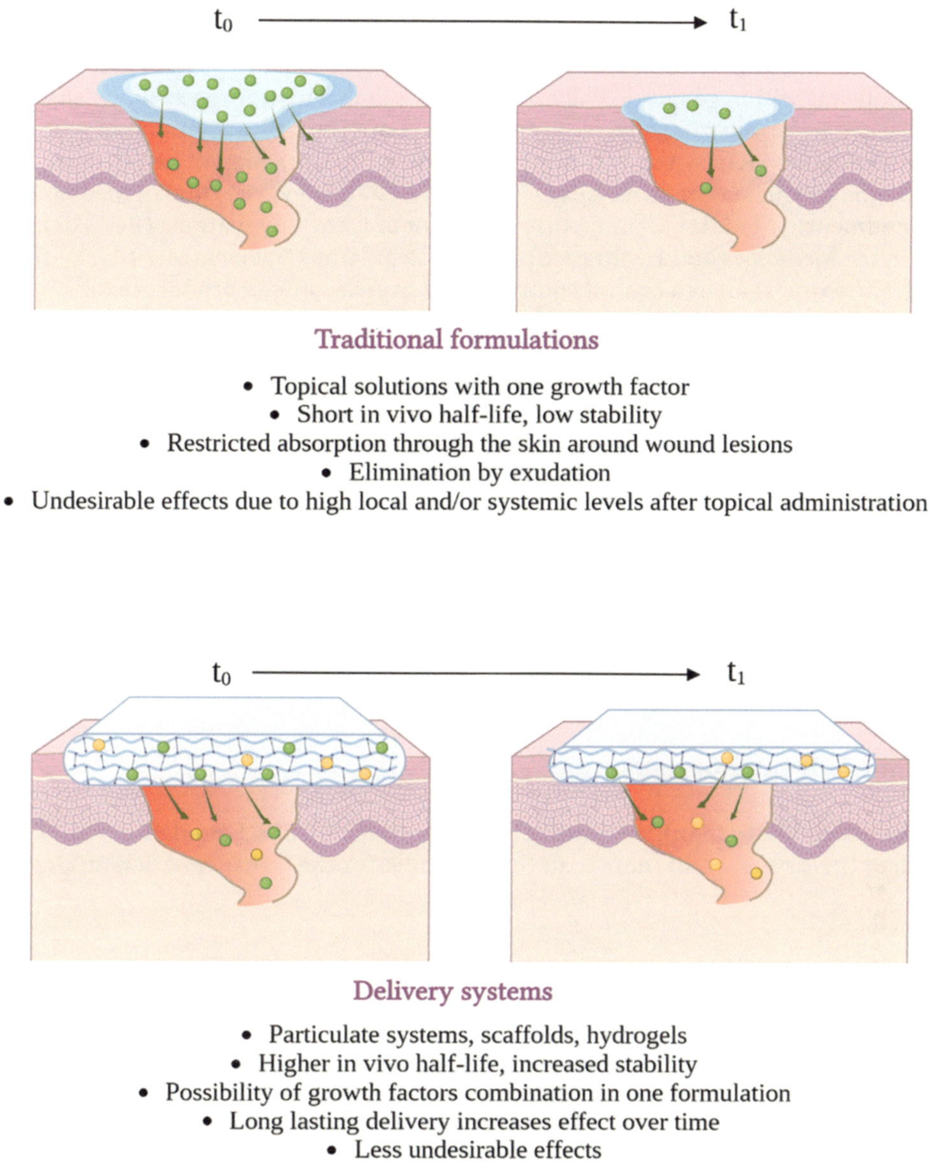

Figure 4.
Traditional formulations generally consist of topical solutions with a single growth factor that has a short half-life and low stability. Absorption is generally limited and necessitates higher doses, which can cause undesired side effects. Improved delivery systems using hydrogels or scaffolds with encapsulation techniques for either traditional pharmaceutics or biologics could improve delivery, increase potential for slow release to augment bioavailability and half-life, and therefore increase stability and lower undesired side effects.

Compliance with legal obligations of appropriate standards and good manufacturing practices (GMP) and good clinical practices (GCP) requires massive work for the management of a clinical study. Global harmonization of procedures could be adapted, as has been recently passed in England for on-site manufacturing at hospitals to increase patient access to medical approaches toward personalized treatments, which could be offered to patients with various pathologies, including oncology, hematology, immunology, rare diseases, and regenerative medicine. This type of policy, just passed in July 2025 in England [101], is forward-thinking, involving expertise available from hospitals to improve rapid care of patients with multidisciplinary teams within geographically restricted regions. This approach allows sharing experience and evaluating adverse events throughout the pathway of manufacture to patient application, which will overall provide an optimization of health care, incite innovation, and improve safety. They have established the Human Medicines (Amendment) (Modular Manufacture and Point of Care) Regulations (POCAR) within the Medicines and Healthcare products Regulatory Agency (MHRA). Within this framework, there is a central control site to oversee on-site production of advanced therapies and other short-shelf-life preparations in hospitals to improve patient care, reduce wait times, and increase security. The legislation covers a variety of advanced products, including cell and gene therapies, 3D-printed treatments, and tissue-engineered products. The overall goal to assure highly personalized and innovative medicines has accelerated access to patients in need but with proportionate control of risks, safety, quality, and efficacy. This new framework retains equivalent levels of safety, quality, and efficacy and is based on a similar concept to that established for blood products and quality control while allowing a necessary flexibility of product type. Based on this extensive guidance, other European countries and Switzerland can aspire to such patient-oriented manufacturing models. Cell therapies and their formulations, which have been standardized, would benefit from point-of-care manufacture and modular manufactured medicinal products.

Acknowledgements

We would like to thank the Sandoz Family Foundation and Foundation S.A.N.T.E. for all of their support for more than three decades for the transplantation program.

Author details

Zhifeng Liao[1], Xi Chen[1], Nathalie Hirt-Burri[1], Alexandre Porcello[2], Cíntia Marques[2], Kelly Lourenço[2], Alexis Laurent[3] and Lee Ann Applegate[1*]

1 Lausanne University Hospital, Epalinges, Switzerland

2 Louna Regenerative SA, Geneva, Switzerland

3 LAM Biotechnologies SA, Epalinges, Switzerland

*Address all correspondence to: lee.laurent-applegate@chuv.ch

References

[1] Wilkinson HN, Hardman MJ. Wound healing: Cellular mechanisms and pathological outcomes. Open Biology. 2020;**10**(9):200223

[2] Fairlamb DM et al. First clinical evaluation of the safety and efficacy of tarumase for the debridement of venous leg ulcers. International Wound Journal. 2024;**21**(3):e14805

[3] Rowlatt U. Intrauterine wound healing in a 20 week human fetus. Virchows Archiv A Pathological Anatomy and Histology. 1979;**381**(3):353-361

[4] Shah M, Foreman DM, Ferguson MW. Control of scarring in adult wounds by neutralising antibody to transforming growth factor beta. Lancet. 1992;**339**(8787):213-214

[5] Lorenz HP et al. Scarless wound repair: A human fetal skin model. Development. 1992;**114**(1):253-259

[6] Lorenz HP, Adzick NS. Scarless skin wound repair in the fetus. The Western Journal of Medicine. 1993;**159**(3):350-355

[7] Longaker MT et al. Adult skin wounds in the fetal environment heal with scar formation. Annals of Surgery. 1994;**219**(1):65-72

[8] Adzick NS, Lorenz HP. Cells, matrix, growth factors, and the surgeon. The biology of scarless fetal wound repair. Annals of Surgery. 1994;**220**(1):10-18

[9] Armstrong JR, Ferguson MW. Ontogeny of the skin and the transition from scar-free to scarring phenotype during wound healing in the pouch young of a marsupial, Monodelphis domestica. Developmental Biology. 1995;**169**(1):242-260

[10] Gomes M et al. Fetal skin wound healing: Key extracellular matrix components and regulators in scarless healing. The Journal of Investigative Dermatology. 2025;**145**(2):280-302

[11] Chen X et al. Bicomponent cutaneous cell therapy for early burn care: Manufacturing homogeneity and epidermis-structuring functions of clinical grade FE002-SK2 allogeneic dermal progenitor fibroblasts. Pharmaceutics. 2025;**17**(6)

[12] Nurkesh A et al. Recent advances in the controlled release of growth factors and cytokines for improving cutaneous wound healing. Frontiers in Cell and Development Biology. 2020;**8**:638

[13] Jimi S et al. Sequential delivery of cryogel released growth factors and cytokines accelerates wound healing and improves tissue regeneration. Frontiers in Bioengineering and Biotechnology. 2020;**8**:345

[14] Pittelkow MR. Growth factors in cutaneous biology and disease. Advances in Dermatology. 1992;**7**:55-81. discussion 82

[15] Fisher DA, Lakshmanan J. Metabolism and effects of epidermal growth factor and related growth factors in mammals. Endocrine Reviews. 1990;**11**(3):418-442

[16] Brown GL et al. Enhancement of wound healing by topical treatment with epidermal growth factor. The New England Journal of Medicine. 1989;**321**(2):76-79

[17] Brown GL et al. Stimulation of healing of chronic wounds by epidermal growth factor. Plastic and Reconstructive Surgery. 1991;**88**(2):189-194. discussion 195-6

[18] Falanga V et al. Topical use of human recombinant epidermal growth factor (h-EGF) in venous ulcers. The Journal of Dermatologic Surgery and Oncology. 1992;**18**(7):604-606

[19] Berlanga-Acosta J et al. Diabetic foot ulcers and epidermal growth factor: Revisiting the local delivery route for a successful outcome. BioMed Research International. 2017;**2017**:2923759

[20] Buckley A et al. Sustained release of epidermal growth factor accelerates wound repair. Proceedings of the National Academy of Sciences of the United States of America. 1985;**82**(21):7340-7344

[21] Acosta JB et al. Epidermal growth factor intralesional infiltrations can prevent amputation in patients with advanced diabetic foot wounds. International Wound Journal. 2006;**3**(3):232-239

[22] Fernandez-Montequin JI et al. Intra-lesional injections of recombinant human epidermal growth factor promote granulation and healing in advanced diabetic foot ulcers: Multicenter, randomised, placebo-controlled, double-blind study. International Wound Journal. 2009;**6**(6):432-443

[23] Gomez-Villa R et al. Efficacy of intralesional recombinant human epidermal growth factor in diabetic foot ulcers in Mexican patients: A randomized double-blinded controlled trial. Wound Repair and Regeneration. 2014;**22**(4):497-503

[24] Hirt-Burri N et al. Wound-healing gene family expression differences between fetal and foreskin cells used for bioengineered skin substitutes. Artificial Organs. 2008;**32**(7):509-518

[25] Wong JK et al. Reduction of tendon adhesions following administration of Adaprev, a hypertonic solution of mannose-6-phosphate: Mechanism of action studies. PLoS One. 2014;**9**(11):e112672

[26] Ferguson MW et al. Prophylactic administration of avotermin for improvement of skin scarring: Three double-blind, placebo-controlled, phase I/II studies. Lancet. 2009;**373**(9671):1264-1274

[27] Occleston NL et al. New therapeutics for the prevention and reduction of scarring. Drug Discovery Today. 2008;**13**(21-22):973-981

[28] Shares in Shire's Partner Renovo Plummet on Clinical Trial Results for Juvista. 2011. Available from: https://firstwordpharma.com/story/1171415

[29] Renovo. Available from: https://pharmaboardroom.com/directory/renovo/

[30] Prevascar in African Continental Group Scarring. Available from: https://clinicaltrials.gov/study/NCT01115868

[31] Rename Plan for Renovo. Available from: https://www.insidermedia.com/news/north-west/119202-rename-plan-renovo

[32] Future Bleak for Renovo with no Workers or Products. Available from: https://pharmatimes.com/news/future_bleak_for_renovo_with_no_workers_or_products_980961/

[33] Rothe MJ, Pesce K, Falanga V. Clinical application of growth factors in cutaneous wound healing. Clinical Immunotherapeutics. 1994;**1**(4):282-292

[34] Senet P. Becaplermin gel (Regranex gel). Annales de Dermatologie et de Vénéréologie. 2004;**131**(4):351-358

[35] REGRANEX(R) Gel 0.01%. Available from: https://www.accessdata.fda.gov/drugsatfda_docs/label/2008/103691s5074lbl.pdf

[36] FDA Approves Removal of Boxed Warning from REGRANEX◊ (becaplermin) gel, 0.01% as Multiple Studies Demonstrate Product Safety. Available from: https://www.smith-nephew.com/news/2018/12/05/20181205-fda-approves-removal-of-boxed-warning-from-regranex-gel

[37] Information Letter regarding Regranex® Gel (becaplermin): Discontinuation of distribution in Europe. Available from: https://www.bfarm.de/SharedDocs/Risikoinformationen/Pharmakovigilanz/EN/RHB/2011/info-regranex.html

[38] Haynes JH et al. Platelet-derived growth factor induces fetal wound fibrosis. Journal of Pediatric Surgery. 1994;**29**(11):1405-1408

[39] Chin GS et al. Differential expression of receptor tyrosine kinases and Shc in fetal and adult rat fibroblasts: Toward defining scarless versus scarring fibroblast phenotypes. Plastic and Reconstructive Surgery. 2000;**105**(3):972-979

[40] Robson MC et al. The safety and effect of topically applied recombinant basic fibroblast growth factor on the healing of chronic pressure sores. Annals of Surgery. 1992;**216**(4):401-406. discussion 406-8

[41] Werner S. Keratinocyte growth factor: A unique player in epithelial repair processes. Cytokine & Growth Factor Reviews. 1998;**9**(2):153-165

[42] Freytes CO et al. Phase I/II randomized trial evaluating the safety and clinical effects of repifermin administered to reduce mucositis in patients undergoing autologous hematopoietic stem cell transplantation. Clinical Cancer Research. 2004;**10**(24):8318-8324

[43] Lee NJ et al. Increased expression of transforming growth factor-beta1, acidic fibroblast growth factor, and basic fibroblast growth factor in fetal versus adult fibroblast cell lines. Laryngoscope. 2000;**110**(4):616-619

[44] The TRAfermin in Neuropathic Diabetic Foot Ulcer Study - Northern Europe The TRANS-North Study (TRANS-North). Available from: https://clinicaltrials.gov/study/NCT01217476

[45] The TRAfermin in Neuropathic Diabetic Foot Ulcer Study - Southern Europe The TRANS-South Study (TRANS-South). Available from: https://www.clinicaltrials.gov/study/NCT01217463

[46] Abdelhakim M, Lin X, Ogawa R. The Japanese experience with basic fibroblast growth factor in cutaneous wound management and scar prevention: A systematic review of clinical and biological aspects. Dermatology Therapy (Heidelberg). 2020;**10**(4):569-587

[47] Matsumoto S et al. The effect of control-released basic fibroblast growth factor in wound healing: Histological analyses and clinical application. Plastic and Reconstructive Surgery. Global Open. 2013;**1**(6):e44

[48] Hayashida K, Akita S. Quality of pediatric second-degree burn wound scars following the application of basic fibroblast growth factor: Results of a randomized, controlled pilot study. Ostomy/Wound Management. 2012;**58**(8):32-36

[49] Hayashida K et al. Effectiveness of basic fibroblast growth factor for pediatric hand burns. Journal of Tissue Viability. 2016;**25**(4):220-224

[50] Hui Q et al. FGF family: From drug development to clinical application. International Journal of Molecular Sciences. 2018;**19**(7)

[51] Fu X et al. Recombinant bovine basic fibroblast growth factor accelerates wound healing in patients with burns, donor sites and chronic dermal ulcers. Chinese Medical Journal. 2000;**113**(4):367-371

[52] Ma B et al. Randomized, multicenter, double-blind, and placebo-controlled trial using topical recombinant human acidic fibroblast growth factor for deep partial-thickness burns and skin graft donor site. Wound Repair and Regeneration. 2007;**15**(6):795-799

[53] Zhang X et al. IGF-1 inhibits inflammation and accelerates angiogenesis via Ras/PI3K/IKK/NF-kappaB signaling pathways to promote wound healing. European Journal of Pharmaceutical Sciences. 2024;**200**:106847

[54] Chaudhari N et al. Topical application of an irreversible small molecule inhibitor of lysyl oxidases ameliorates skin scarring and fibrosis. Nature Communications. 2022;**13**(1):5555

[55] Medsger TA Jr et al. D-penicillamine in systemic sclerosis? Yes! Scandinavian Journal of Rheumatology. 2001;**30**(4):192-194

[56] Ren M et al. Connective tissue growth factor: Regulation, diseases, and drug discovery. International Journal of Molecular Sciences. 2024;**25**(9)

[57] Obeng MK et al. Cadaveric allograft discards as a result of positive skin cultures. Burns. 2001;**27**(3):267-271

[58] Parcells AL et al. The use of fetal bovine dermal scaffold (PriMatrix) in the management of full-thickness hand burns. Eplasty. 2014;**14**:e36

[59] Sun BK, Siprashvili Z, Khavari PA. Advances in skin grafting and treatment of cutaneous wounds. Science. 2014;**346**(6212):941-945

[60] Monavarian M et al. Regenerative scar-free skin wound healing. Tissue Engineering Part B, Reviews. 2019;**25**(4):294-311

[61] Cerceo JR et al. Management of large full-thickness burns using kerecis acellular fish skin graft and recell autologous skin cell suspension: A case report of two patients with large surface area burns. Cureus. 2024;**16**(10):e71101

[62] Mukherjee S et al. Application of tilapia fish skin in treatment of burn patients. Biocatalysis and Agricultural Biotechnology. 2024;**59**:103254

[63] Philandrianos C et al. Comparison of five dermal substitutes in full-thickness skin wound healing in a porcine model. Burns. 2012;**38**(6):820-829

[64] Russo B, Brembilla NC, Chizzolini C. Interplay between keratinocytes and fibroblasts: A systematic review providing a new angle for understanding skin fibrotic disorders. Frontiers in Immunology. 2020;**11**:648

[65] Goedkoop R et al. Wound stimulation by growth-arrested human keratinocytes and fibroblasts: HP802-247, a new-generation allogeneic tissue engineering product. Dermatology. 2010;**220**(2):114-120

[66] Feisst V et al. Rapid culture of human keratinocytes in an autologous, feeder-free system with a novel growth medium. Cytotherapy. 2023;**25**(2):174-184

[67] Ghio SC et al. A newly developed chemically defined serum-free medium suitable for human primary keratinocyte culture and tissue engineering applications. International Journal of Molecular Sciences. 2023;**24**(3)

[68] Varkey M, Ding J, Tredget EE. Superficial dermal fibroblasts enhance basement membrane and epidermal barrier formation in tissue-engineered skin: Implications for treatment of skin basement membrane disorders. Tissue Engineering Part A. 2014;**20**(3-4):540-552

[69] White P et al. Deletion of the homeobox gene PRX-2 affects fetal but not adult fibroblast wound healing responses. The Journal of Investigative Dermatology. 2003;**120**(1):135-144

[70] Rangatchew F et al. Mesenchymal stem cell therapy of acute thermal burns: A systematic review of the effect on inflammation and wound healing. Burns. 2021;**47**(2):270-294

[71] Qiao Y et al. Effect of stem cell treatment on burn wounds: A systemic review and a meta-analysis. International Wound Journal. 2023;**20**(1):8-17

[72] Abdul Kareem N, Aijaz A, Jeschke MG. Stem cell therapy for burns: Story so far. Biologics. 2021;**15**:379-397

[73] Arno A et al. Stem cell therapy: A new treatment for burns? Pharmaceuticals (Basel). 2011;**4**(10):1355-1380

[74] Wang M et al. Mesenchymal stem cell-based therapy for burn wound healing. Burns Trauma. 2021;**9**:tkab002

[75] Wood FM, Kolybaba ML, Allen P. The use of cultured epithelial autograft in the treatment of major burn wounds: Eleven years of clinical experience. Burns. 2006;**32**(5):538-544

[76] Chemali M et al. Burn center organization and cellular therapy integration: Managing risks and costs. Journal of Burn Care & Research. 2021;**42**(5):911-924

[77] MacNeil S. Progress and opportunities for tissue-engineered skin. Nature. 2007;**445**(7130):874-880

[78] Cirodde A et al. Cultured epithelial autografts in massive burns: A single-center retrospective study with 63 patients. Burns. 2011;**37**(6):964-972

[79] Auxenfans C et al. Cultured autologous keratinocytes in the treatment of large and deep burns: A retrospective study over 15 years. Burns. 2015;**41**(1):71-79

[80] Ter Horst B et al. Advances in keratinocyte delivery in burn wound care. Advanced Drug Delivery Reviews. 2018;**123**:18-32

[81] Esteban-Vives R et al. Cell-spray auto-grafting technology for deep partial-thickness burns: Problems and solutions during clinical implementation. Burns. 2018;**44**(3):549-559

[82] Chen X et al. Cutaneous cell therapy manufacturing timeframe rationalization: Allogeneic off-the-freezer fibroblasts for dermo-epidermal combined preparations (DE-FE002-SK2) in burn care. Pharmaceutics. 2023;**15**(9)

[83] Nilforoushzadeh MA et al. Application of dermal fibroblast cells in cell therapy of wound. Journal of Skin and Stem Cell. 2017;**4**(3-4):1-6

[84] Rheinwald JG, Green H. Serial cultivation of strains of human epidermal keratinocytes: The formation of keratinizing colonies from single cells. Cell. 1975;**6**(3):331-343

[85] Hartmann B et al. Sprayed cultured epithelial autografts for deep dermal burns of the face and neck. Annals of Plastic Surgery. 2007;**58**(1):70-73

[86] Sabeh G et al. New process: Do sequential skin cell transplants cure third degree burns? Comparative study on 517 patients. Annals of Burns and Fire Disasters. 2018;**31**(3):213-222

[87] Kirsner RS et al. Spray-applied cell therapy with human allogeneic fibroblasts and keratinocytes for the treatment of chronic venous leg ulcers: A phase 2, multicentre, double-blind, randomised, placebo-controlled trial. Lancet. 2012;**380**(9846):977-985

[88] Healiva Acquires B. Braun's Cell Therapy Manufacturing Assets. Available from: https://www.mpo-mag.com/breaking-news/healiva-acquires-b-brauns-cell-therapy-manufacturing-assets/

[89] Yim H et al. A clinical trial designed to evaluate the safety and effectiveness of a thermosensitive hydrogel-type cultured epidermal allograft for deep second-degree burns. Burns. 2014;**40**(8):1642-1649

[90] Kim EH, Lee SH. Efficacy of cultured allogenic keratinocytes in treatment of deep second-degree burn. Journal of Burn Care & Research. 2021;**42**(3):533-537

[91] Wood FM et al. Characterisation of the cell suspension harvested from the dermal epidermal junction using a ReCell(R) kit. Burns. 2012;**38**(1):44-51

[92] Bolivar-Flores YJ, Kuri-Harcuch W. Frozen allogeneic human epidermal cultured sheets for the cure of complicated leg ulcers. Dermatologic Surgery. 1999;**25**(8):610-617

[93] Quintin A et al. Consistency and safety of cell banks for research and clinical use: Preliminary analysis of fetal skin banks. Cell Transplantation. 2007;**16**(7):675-684

[94] Flahaut M et al. Reassessing long-term cryopreservation strategies for improved quality, safety, and clinical use of allogeneic dermal progenitor cells. The Journal of Investigative Dermatology. 2024;**144**(10):2125-2135

[95] Al-Dourobi K et al. Retrospective evaluation of progenitor biological bandage use: A complementary and safe therapeutic management option for prevention of hypertrophic scarring in pediatric burn care. Pharmaceuticals (Basel). 2021;**14**(3)

[96] Xue M et al. Dermal fibroblast heterogeneity and its contribution to the skin repair and regeneration. Advances in Wound Care (New Rochelle). 2022;**11**(2):87-107

[97] Bisson F et al. Irradiated human dermal fibroblasts are as efficient as mouse fibroblasts as a feeder layer to improve human epidermal cell culture lifespan. International Journal of Molecular Sciences. 2013;**14**(3):4684-4704

[98] Lenihan C et al. The effect of isolation and culture methods on epithelial stem cell populations and their progeny-toward an improved cell expansion protocol for clinical application. Cytotherapy. 2014;**16**(12):1750-1759

[99] Kathju S, Gallo PH, Satish L. Scarless integumentary wound healing in the

mammalian fetus: Molecular basis and therapeutic implications. Birth Defects Research Part C, Embryo Today. 2012;**96**(3):223-236

[100] Scar Treatment Market To Generate $52.8 Billion Revenue by 2030. Available from: https://www.psmarketresearch.com/press-release/global-scar-treatment-market

[101] Available from: https://www.gov.uk/government/publications/human-medicines-modular-manufacture-and-point-of-care-regulations-2025-overview/human-medicines-modular-manufacture-and-point-of-care-regulations-2025-overview [Accessed: September 1, 2025]

Chapter 7

Tissue Engineering for Wound Healing

Arzu Dinç Yavaş

Abstract

Wounds represent a serious clinical problem for patients and clinicians. Wound healing process involves interaction between the extracellular matrix (ECM) and cells, including fibroblasts, keratinocytes, endothelial cells, macrophages, and platelets. Growth factors (GFs), cytokines, and chemokines are also the important factors. Defects in one of the steps of the process can lead to wound healing impairment. Various treatment techniques have been used to enhance the wound healing process. Tissue engineering is the combination of methods that promote biologic regeneration or repair of tissues by providing signaling, structural, or tissue replacement functions through systems that contain living tissue or cells. Biomaterials, cells, growth factors, other signaling molecules, and engineering components, such as scaffolds, pumps, tubes, bioreactors, and oxygenators, are the main elements of tissue engineering. The major principle of tissue engineering is to restore and improve the function of the tissues by either generating novel or biocompatible substitutes or by reconstructing the tissues.

Keywords: wound, tissue, scaffold, biomaterial, regeneration

1. Introduction

Wound healing process involves interaction between the extracellular matrix (ECM) and cells, including fibroblasts, keratinocytes, endothelial cells, macrophages, and platelets [1, 2]. Growth factors (GFs), cytokines, and chemokines are also the important factors. Defects in one of the steps of the process can lead to wound healing impairment [2].

The aim of this chapter is to explore wound treatment options using tissue engineering. Repair of tissues is achieved by supporting the tissue functions with systems that contain biomaterials, cells, growth factors, other signaling molecules, and engineering components, such as scaffolds, pumps, tubes, bioreactors, and oxygenators, which are the study areas of tissue engineering [3].

2. Tissue engineering in wound treatment

2.1 Biomaterials

Scaffolds are the best materials to restore, maintain, and improve tissue function [4]. Desired properties of biomaterials for use in wound healing are mechanical strength, flexibility, porosity, structure, biodegradability, and biocompatibility [5]. The wright biomaterial must promote cell survival. Cells need to proliferate and differentiate in an appropriate biomaterial for tissue regeneration [6]. The term mechanical strength defines the fracture resistance, load bearing capacity, and structural integrity, capability of keeping the same shape against tensile forces. Flexibility is to conform to the wound's shape. These are especially important because for wound treatment, biomaterials must be tailored according to the lesion location, size, and depth. Porosity is important for oxygen and nutrient diffusion, cell infiltration, and disposal of the wastes. Structural properties (microarchitecture, interconnectivity, hydrophobicity/hydrophilicity), and biodegradability (breakdown of the biomaterial to harmless components) and biocompatibilty (proper interaction of the biomaterial with natural tissues without causing harmful effects) are other desired properties of biomaterials [6].

Tissue engineering uses biomaterials, such as scaffolds, films, foams, hydrocolloids, and hydrogels (**Figure 1**). These may be synthetic or natural and degradable or non-degradable [7]. Collagen, silk, gelatin, and fibrinogen are natural biomaterials used in tissue engineering [5]. Composite biomaterials combine two or more different types of materials, each with distinct properties. Cellulose and chitosan nanoparticles combined with cellulose polymethylmethacrylate fibers is an example of a composite biomaterial used in wound healing [5]. Synthetic biomaterials such as polyglycolic acid (PGA), polylactic acid (PLA) and their copolymers, polyethylene glycol (PEG), and poly-b-hydroxybutyrate (PHB), have desired properties (e.g. porosity, degradation time and mechanical characteristics) and could be tailored for the specific applications [8]. These are polyhydroxyl ortho esters [8].

2.1.1 Natural biomaterials

Natural biomaterials' structure resembles to the extracellular matrix (ECM); this property makes them an ideal scaffold for tissue repair (5).

2.1.1.1 Collagen (col)

Collagen is the major protein of the extracellular matrix (ECM) that can be originated from nature (bovine human collagen, rooster neck, eggshell membrane, marine creatures) or vegetables [9].

Collagen can also be produced by recombinant methods [10]. Mechanical and hydrophilic properties and degradation of collagen-based scaffolds can be customized by changing the concentrations of collagen and glycosaminoglycan compositions [11, 12]. Difficulty in sterilization and degradation are major limitations [13]. Collagen has importance in inflammation, debridement, angiogenesis, and re-epithelialization of wound healing [14].

The effect of collagen in wound healing depends on the hemostatic effect, interaction with fibronectin, and platelets. It enhances fibroblast production and permeation, and inhibits the matrix degrading enzymes. Fibronectin plays a key role in cell cycle succession, cell endurance, and divergence [14, 15].

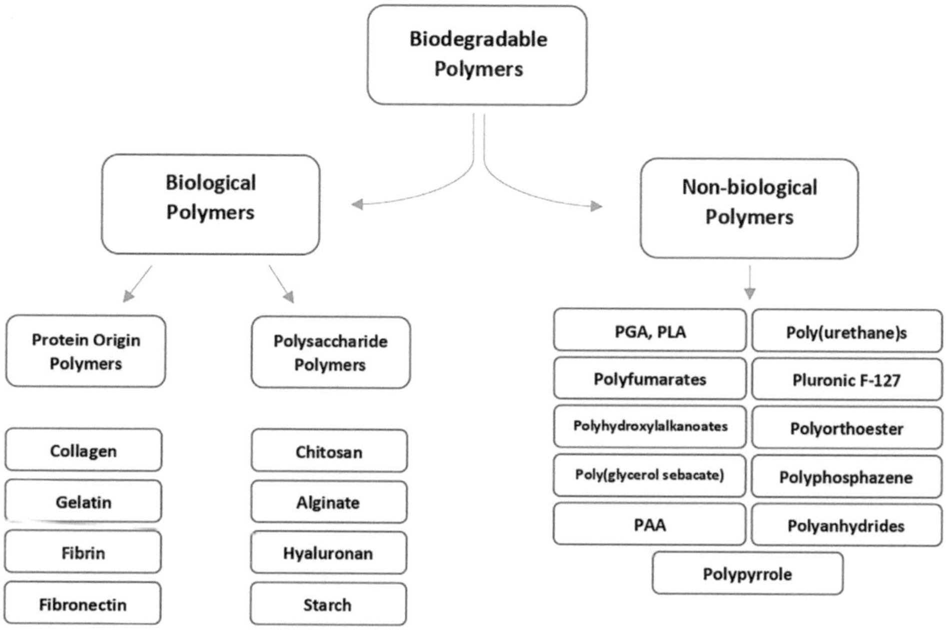

Figure 1.
Components of tissue engineering.

Apligraf R is a bilayered collagen scaffold, including human fibroblasts as the "dermal" matrix and human keratinocytes as epidermal layer [16]. Biomed VR is a collagen membrane that commonly used in the periodontal tissue regeneration [12]. Integra is a bovine collagen-based bilaminate membrane of glycosaminoglycans and chondroitin-6-sulphate and a temporary epidermal substitute layer of semipermeable silicone product used to treat burns [17–19].

2.1.1.2 Cellulose

Cellulose is a type of polysaccharide with high capability to retain water and maintain its mechanical strength, and its similarity to ECM has attracted great potential, but biodegradability problems are challenging for its use [20, 21]. The combination of bacterial cellulose and human urine-derived stem cells showed better results in terms of wound healing [20].

2.1.1.3 Silk

Silk is one of the natural biomaterials consisting of fibroin and sericin proteins. Biocompatible and biodegradable fibroin protein has low immunogenicity and upregulates transcription factor nuclear factor kappa-B (NF-kB), which has a major role in wound healing process [22]. Sericin protein has been shown to enhance tissue regeneration [23, 24].

2.1.1.4 Fibrin

Fibrinogen is a plasma protein and a precursor of fibrin, which is important for cell adhesion. Fibrin gels release growth factors, cytokines, or other bioactive molecules. Fibrin gel alone or as a scaffold combined with other tissue factors is used in wound healing. Fibrin scaffolds can be modified according to fibrin content [25].

2.1.1.5 Fibronectin

Fibronectin is a high molecular weight plasma glycoprotein, which can bind collagen, fibrin, and heparin, and participates in the wound healing procedure [26].

2.1.1.6 Gelatine

Gelatine is derived from collagen and has variable flexibility under appropriate temperature and pH [27]. Gelatin-alginate sponges, gelatin-containing epidermal growth factor (EGF), and gelatin films have been used [5]. Gelatin has lower immunogenicity and greater cellular adhesion potential than collagen [28].

2.1.1.7 Elastin

Elastin is an insoluble and hydrophobic protein combined with collagen and produced by electrospinning technology as a scaffold for dermal tissue engineering [29].

2.1.1.8 Chitosan

Chitosan is a biodegradable natural polysaccharide and has a strong tissue-adhesive property with an enhanced blood coagulation [30, 31]. Chitosan promotes collagen and hyaluronic acid synthesis, and migration of inflammatory cells into the wound site; also, it has microbicidal activity [32–35].

2.1.1.9 Keratin

Keratin is the main structural fibrous protein of skin, which has promising results for wound healing [36, 37].

2.1.1.10 Alginate

Alginate dressing Kaltostat stimulates the monocytes to produce cytokines, such as interleukin-6 and tumor necrosis factor-α, which are the main factors in wound healing [38]. Alginate alone or in combination with chitosan and collagen can be used as a skin substitute [39].

2.1.1.11 Hyaluronic acid (hyaluronan)

Hyaluronic acid (HA) is a glycosaminoglycan, which can be used as a topical agent in the treatment of burns and skin ulcers [40].

2.1.2 Synthetic biomaterials

PLA/PGA-combined scaffolds are ideal for internal fixation because of slow degradation rate and constant transfer of loads to the tissues [41]. They are used as drug delivery systems to treat infected wounds [42, 43].

2.1.2.1 Polylactic acid (PLA)

PLA fibrous membranes (PFMs) have been used in a study to release bioactive molecules for tissue repair [44]. The H2S-releasing PFMs are found to be a cost-effective and efficient scaffold for tissue repair. In another study, PLA was reported as a delivery system for treating oral mucosal diseases [45].

2.1.2.2 Polyglycolic acid (PGA)

PGA consists of repeating glycolic acid units. Kibe et al. studied PGA wound dressing in rats with full-thickness defects and found that PGA is superior to collagen-based wound dressing in controlling the exhibition of alpha-smooth muscle actin.

Alpha SMA can be linked to increased fibrosis and scar contracture [46].

2.1.2.3 Polyethylene oxide

Polyethylene oxide and chitosan-composed nanofiber mesh have been used to treat full-thickness skin wounds of rats in order to distribute growth factors, such as vascular endothelial growth factor (VEGF) and platelet-derived growth factor BB (PDGF-BB), which are important in angiogenesis and tissue remodeling, and regeneration by earlier deposition of collagen [47].

2.1.2.4 Polyethylene glycol

Polyethylene glycol (PEG) has low immune response and also protects the cells from damage [48].

2.1.2.5 Poly-b-hydroxybutyrate

The efficacy of poly-b-hydroxybutyrate (PHB) scaffold loaded with stem cells is reported for the treatment of the acute full-thickness skin wounds [49].

2.1.2.6 Poly(vinyl alcohol)

PVA and chitosan blends were produced by electrospinning for wound treatment [50].

2.1.2.7 Polycaprolactone

Polycaprolactone (PCL) scaffolds loaded with stem cells have promising effects in healing skin defects [51]. Hou *et al.* [52] created a sandwich-structured scaffold with a polycaprolactone (PCL) nanofiber core and collagen with N-acetylcysteine (NAC) effective in full-thickness skin defect wound models. It showed increased angiogenesis and enhanced epidermal maturation after 21 days.

2.1.3 Hybrid scaffolds

Synthetic biodegradable polymers have good mechanical strength and their degradation periods could also be manipulated by controlling the crystallinity, molecular weight, and copolymer ratio, but they lack cell recognition signals, and they do not provide a suitable environment for smooth cell seeding [53–55]. Therefore, scaffolds containing natural and synthetic polymers were hybridized to combine the advantageous properties of both constitutes [56].

2.2 Skin substitutes

Early and proper healing of wound without contracture and scar formation, and ideally regeneration of the skin are the signs of a successfully treated wound. Dermal substitutes play a crucial role in reducing scar formation in skin reconstruction, inhibiting excessive proliferation and improving softness and contracture, as well as improving mechanical wear resistance [57].

2.2.1 Acellular skin substitutes

Human- or animal-tissue-derived acellular substitutes, or immunogenic cellular components, are removed using decellularization techniques [44]. Decellularizing the ECM may help address the wound site problems, such as oxidative stress and biofilm formation seen in cellular skin substitutes [58]. Decellularized skin/adipose flaps (DSAFs) composed of collagen and laminin, and supplemented with vascular endothelial growth factors (VEGFs) and basic fibroblast growth factors (FGFs), have been transplanted onto nude rats, resulting in an increase in M2 macrophages and improvement in wound healing [59]. Also, adding media, including secretomes of stem cells to biomaterials in order to increase vascularization for the manufacturing of acellular skin substitutes, is another method of tissue engineering [60, 61].

Integra® is an acellular substitute composed of a collagen/glycosaminoglycan matrix, providing a suitable environment for the dermis cells to grow and a silicone membrane acting as an epidermis, created for patients with severe full-thickness burn injuries [62].

AlloDerm ® is derived from cadaver human dermis preserved by freeze-drying. The removal of cells from AlloDerm reduces the risk of rejection. The decellularized ECM acts as a scaffold containing collagen and elastic fibers, and it allows the regeneration of a new dermis [63].

2.2.2 Cellular skin substitutes and stem cells

In recent years, tissue engineering focused on cellular skin substitutes and stem cells [64]. Stem cells (SC) have self-renewal capacity and multi-lineage differentiation potential. Optimal stem cell starts proliferation, differentiation, and tissue remodeling in the scaffold (**Figure 2**). Types of cells used in tissue engineering are embryonic stem cells (ESCs), induced pluripotent stem cells (iPSCs), fetal stem cells (umbilical cord-derived MSCs, Wharton's jelly MSCs, and human umbilical cord perivascular cells), and adult stem cells (adipose-derived mesenchymal stem cells (ADSCs), bone-marrow-derived mesenchymal stem cells (BM-MSCs), hair follicle stem cells (HFSCs), melanocyte stem cells (MelSCs), fibroblasts, and keratinocytes) [65].

Induced pluripotent stem cells (iPSCs) can differentiate to any desired cell type [66]. In vitro and in vivo studies on mouse models have demonstrated the potential of iPSCs cells in generating a number of human autologous cells for advanced chronic wound treatment and degenerative skin disorders [66–69].

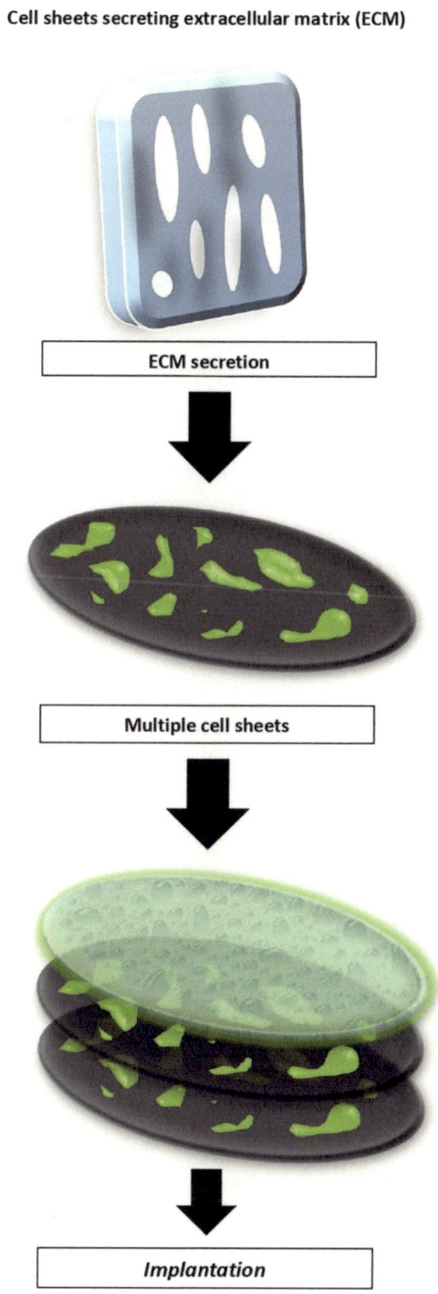

Figure 2.
Cellular skin substitutes.

Hair follicle stem cells (HFSCs), melanocyte stem cells (MelSCs), adipose-derived stem cells (ADSCs), fibroblasts, and keratinocytes are all present in the skin as cell sources for skin healing [70–72].

Hair follicle stem cells (HFSCs) have the ability to differentiate into epidermal cells and sebaceous glands along with other hair cells, and they promote the growth of tissue, regulate inflammation, and accelerate the formation of new blood vessels [72].

ADSCs are mesenchymal stem cells and release GFs important in skin regeneration [71].

Exosomes are mesenchymal stem cell-originated extracellular vesicles containing proteins, which have effects in reducing inflammation and scar tissue in wound healing [73].

Fibroblasts and keratinocytes are the primary sources of dermal substitute production. Dermal fibroblasts are responsible for the synthesis of collagen, elastin, laminin, and glycosaminoglycan; these are structural components of ECM. Epidermal keratinocytes are important for epidermal regeneration. According to the desired treatment effect, keratinocyte or fibroblast-based constructs can be used for dermal regeneration [74]. When applied to the wound site, these cells provide signal molecules, growth factors, and extracellular matrix proteins, supporting skin tissue regeneration [74–76].

Dermagraft® is an absorbable polymer scaffold seeded with neonatal allogeneic fibroblasts. An ECM consisting of collagens, tenascin, vitronectin, glycosaminoglycans, and growth factors is laid down by the fibroblasts and has been used to stimulate wound healing in chronic wounds, such as diabetic foot ulcers, than resurface full-thickness acute burn wounds [74].

2.2.3 Cultured epidermal autografts (CEAs)

CEA is a method to transplant the patient's own keratinocytes obtained from skin biopsy as an epidermal sheet. CEA Epicel® is a technology in which cells are cultured over a period of 3 weeks until thin sheets of keratinocytes are available for grafting [75].

Apligraf® is a bilayered bioengineered skin substitute and provides both cells and a matrix, producing cytokines and growth factors; however, its exact mechanism of action is still unknown [76].

Adipose-derived stem cells (ADSCs) have the ability to promote the proliferation and migration of human dermal fibroblasts (HDFs) through cell-to-cell interactions and paracrine activation on acute wounds [77].

2.2.4 Cultured skin substitutes

Cultured skin substitutes (CSSs) consist of autologous keratinocytes, fibroblasts, and stem cells combined with a bovine collagen matrix, cells secrete GFs, and cytokines to stimulate tissue growth repair [78].

2.2.5 Allogenic skin substitute

Allogenic skin substitutes include fibroblasts and are used for covering wounds temporarily [79].

2.3 3D bioprinting in skin tissue engineering

The use of traditional scaffolds has some limitations: the vascularization of engineered tissues; correct and precise cell deposition in the scaffold; and the stiffness of the support matrix and inflammation due to degradation. Three-dimensional bioprinting processes include magnetic bioprinting, stereolithography, photolithography, and direct cell extrusion. Cells are obtained from the patient and then are suspended in culture media and in a biomaterial solution. This bioink is then printed and incubated in a bioreactor, ensuring proper nutrients and gas flow to get a functional tissue (**Figure 3**) [80].

Bioprinted skin is not the same as natural skin because bioink cannot fully replicate the ECM [81, 82]. Therefore, endothelial progenitor cells and ADSCs added to skin-derived ECM (S-dECM) bioink are used to print a full-thickness 3D human skin model [83]. 3D bioprinted hydrogel scaffolds containing adipose-derived mesenchymal stem cells (ADSCs) and nitric oxide (NO) promote epithelialization, collagen deposition, and neovascularization, contributing to wound healing [84].

Sodium alginate (SA), gellan gum (GG), and polydopamine nanoparticles (PDA NPs) combined bioink was used to print a scaffold for wound healing. The printed

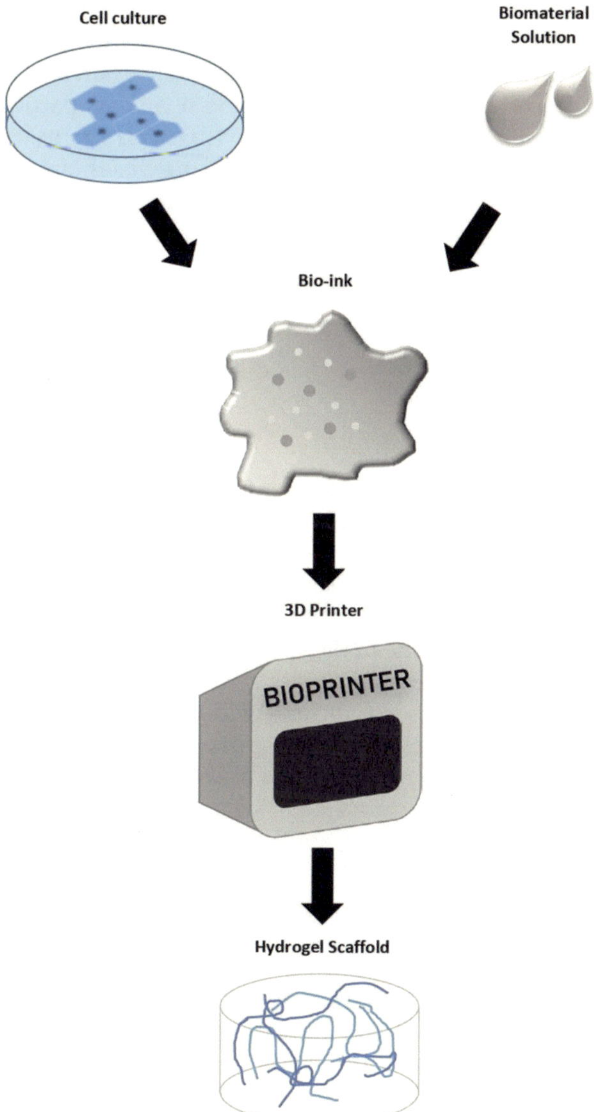

Figure 3.
Bioprinting for tissue engineering.

porous hydrogel scaffold promoted wound healing by enhancing collagen deposition and encouraging proliferation, migration, and tissue ingrowth [85, 86].

3D-printed alginate/gelatin-based porous hydrogel scaffold was found to integrate well with the tissues, promote angiogenesis, and exhibit high levels of collagen deposition, resulting in the healing of diabetic wounds [86].

2.4 Electrospun scaffolds

Electrospinning is a simple and flexible process for fabricating polymer nanofibers. Electrospun scaffolds have variable pore size, high surface area, and oxygen permeability. Bioactive substances, such as growth factors, nanoparticles, antimicrobials, anti-inflammatory agents, and wound healing drugs, can be loaded on electrospun scaffolds [87, 88].

Metal oxide nanoparticles are well known for their antibacterial activities. Silver (AgNPs) nanoparticles inhibit the growth of *Staphylococcus epidermidis* and *Staphylococcus haemolyticus*, and electrospun membranes containing silver nanoparticles have microbicidal activity against gram-positive and gram-negative bacteria strains [89].

Gold nanoparticles have antioxidant effects and are beneficial for wound repair [90]. PCL/gelatin scaffolds containing 6-aminopenicillanic acid (APA) and gold nanoparticles (Au-APA) were reported effective for the treatment of multidrug-resistant bacteria infections [91].

Polyurethane (PU) electrospun scaffolds containing ampicillin has antibacterial properties against *Staphylococcus aureus* and *Klebsiella pneumoniae* [92].

3. Discussion

Recent knowledge about wound treatment has highlighted tissue engineering.

Tissue engineering offers treatments using different types of scaffolds, cell therapy, growth factors, and bioactive molecules.

Embryonic stem cells, iPSCs, and mesenchymal stem cells are currently popular for wound treatment without the risk of immune rejection [93, 94].

Much research needs to be done in the field of hiPSCs in terms of the reprogramming process [95, 96]. MSC therapy provides unique and effective support for stimulating the wound healing process in a chronic wound since these cells have the ability to suppress excessive inflammation and reduce scarring, promoting angiogenesis in the wound [97]. Further studies are necessary to characterize the niche of MSCs to be effective in the wound healing process [94]. The use of stem cells has the potential risks of malignant teratoma formation, and long-term adverse effects of the stem cells should be investigated in this regard [98]. In addition, there is a lack of information on long-term outcomes of skin wound treatment using regenerative therapies.

The other important actors in tissue engineering are scaffolds. The primary challenge in scaffold manufacturing is ensuring the biocompatibility, biodegradability, and integration with the tissues, reducing the risk of immune response or toxicity. Degradation rate of the scaffold must be close to the tissue regeneration process [99]. The scaffold should be flexible and hydrophilic for optimal cell attachment and proliferation in epidermal wounds. Also, scaffolds should promote angiogenesis and have sufficient elasticity to accommodate movement for subcutaneous wounds. Infection is one of the problems for chronic wounds; therefore, the scaffold must have antimicrobial properties or be loaded with antimicrobial agents [99]. Researchers are studying on the nanoscale drug delivery systems that could offer improved compatibility with drug delivery techniques [47].

Emergent technologies for scaffold manufacturing are electrospinning and 3D bioprinting [100, 101]. The structure of electrospun sheets resembles the native ECM architecture, with optimal biomechanical properties. Growth factors, antimicrobials, anti-inflammatory, and antifibrotic agents and drugs promoting wound healing can be incorporated into electrospun scaffolds. 3D bioprinting can help to customize the biomaterials according to the desired wound shape [100]. New challenge in 3D bioprinting improvement is to provide bioinks suitable for different types of cells [101].

Advanced mechanical features, advanced drug delivery capability, advanced biodegradability, and optimized cellular delivery to induce more re-epithelialization are the treatment targets [102].

4. Conclusions

All these types of approaches adopted by regenerative medicine can be enclosed in the technologies offered by tissue engineering. Treating chronic and deep wounds remains a persistent challenge. Continued research and innovation in this field has the potential for wound healing therapies, leading to faster recovery and better wound closure.

Conflict of interest

The authors declare no conflict of interest.

Author details

Arzu Dinç Yavaş[1,2]

1 İstanbul Aydın University School of Medicine, Turkey

2 İstinye University Stem Cell and Tissue Engineering PhD, İstanbul, Turkey

*Address all correspondence to: arzu.dinc@aydin.edu.tr

References

[1] Barrientos S, Stojadinovic O, Golinko MS, Brem H, Tomic-Canic M. Growth factors and cytokines in wound healing. Wound Repair and Regeneration. 2008;**16**:585-601

[2] Wilkinson HN, Hardman MJ. Wound healing: Cellular mechanisms and pathological outcomes. Open Biology. 2020;**10**:200223

[3] Ehrenreich M, Ruszczak Z. Update on tissue-engineered biological dressings. Tissue Engineering. 2006;**12**:2407-2424

[4] O'Brien FJ. Biomaterials & scaffolds for tissue engineering. Materials Today. 2011;**14**:88-95

[5] Chaudhari AA, Vig K, Baganizi DR, Sahu R, Dixit S, Dennis V, et al. Future prospects for scaffolding methods and biomaterials in skin tissue engineering: A review. International Journal of Molecular Sciences. 1974;**2016**:17

[6] Niculescu AG, Grumezescu AM. An up-to-date review of biomaterials application in wound management. Polymers. 2022;**14**:421

[7] Nair LS, Laurencin CT. Biodegradable polymers as biomaterials. Progress in Polymer Science. 2007;**32**:762-798

[8] Rahmani Del Bakhshayesh A, Annabi N, Khalilov R, Akbarzadeh A, Samiei M, Alizadeh E, et al. Recent advances on biomedical applications of scaffolds in wound healing and dermal tissue engineering. Artificial Cells, Nanomedicine, and Biotechnology. 2017;**46**(4):691-705. DOI: 10.1080/21691401.2017.1349778

[9] Avila Rodríguez MI, Rodriguez Barroso LG, Sánchez ML. Collagen: A review on its sources and potential cosmetic applications. Journal of Cosmetic Dermatology. 2018;**17**(1):20-26

[10] Massia SP, Holecko MM, Ehteshami GR. In vitro assessment of bioactive coatings for neural implant applications. Journal of Biomedical Materials Research. Part A. 2004;**68**:177-186

[11] McKinney L, Hollinger JO. A bone regeneration study: Transforming growth factor-[beta] 1 and its delivery. The Journal of Craniofacial Surgery. 1996;7:36-45

[12] Burke JF, Yannas IV, Quinby WC Jr, et al. Successful use of a physiologically acceptable artificial skin in the treatment of extensive burn injury. Annals of Surgery. 1981;**194**:413

[13] Brett D. A review of collagen and collagen-based wound dressings. Wounds. 2008;**20**(12):347-356

[14] Hochstein AO, Bhatia A. Collagen: Its role in wound healing. Wound Management. 2014;**4**(1):104-109

[15] Huang S, Deng T, Wang Y, et al. Multifunctional implantable particles for skin tissue regeneration: Preparation, characterization, in vitro and in vivo studies. Acta Biomaterialia. 2008;**4**:1057-1066

[16] Danielsson C, Ruault S, Basset-Dardare A, et al. Modified collagen fleece, a scaffold for transplantation of human bladder smooth muscle cells. Biomaterials. 2006;**27**:1054-1060

[17] Fitton AR, Drew P, Dickson WA. The use of a bilaminate artificialskin substitute (Integra^{TM}) in acute

resurfacing of burns: An early experience. British Journal of Plastic Surgery. 2001;**54**:208-212

[18] Heimbach DM, Warden GD, Luterman A, et al. Multicenter postapproval clinical trial of IntegraVR dermal regeneration template for burn treatment. Journal of Burn Care & Research. 2003;**24**:42-48

[19] Li M, Han M, Sun Y, Hua Y, Chen G, Zhang L. Oligoarginine mediated collagen/chitosan gel composite for cutaneous wound healing. International Journal of Biological Macromolecules. 2019;**122**:1120-1127

[20] Cao YM, Liu MY, Xue ZW, Qiu Y, Li J, Wang Y, et al. Surface-structured bacterial cellulose loaded with hUSCs accelerate skin wound healing by promoting angiogenesis in rats. Biochemical and Biophysical Research Communications. 2019;**516**:1167-1174

[21] Park YR, Sultan MT, Park HJ, Lee JM, Ju HW, Lee OJ, et al. NF-κB signaling is key in the wound healing processes of silk fibroin. Acta Biomaterialia. 2018;**67**:183-195

[22] Chouhan D, Mandal BB. Silk biomaterials in wound healing and skin regeneration therapeutics: From bench to bedside. Acta Biomaterialia. 2020;**103**:24-51

[23] Mazurek Ł, Szudzik M, Rybka M, Konop M. Silk fibroin biomaterials and their beneficial role in skin wound healing. Biomolecules. 2022;**12**:1852

[24] Napavichayanun S, Ampawong S, Harnsilpong T, Angspatt A, Aramwit P. Inflammatory reaction, clinical efficacy, and safety of bacterial cellulose wound dressing containing silk sericin and polyhexamethylene biguanide for wound treatment. Archives of Dermatological Research. 2018;**310**(10):795-805. DOI: 10.1007/s00403-018-1871-3. Epub 2018 Oct 9

[25] Herbert CB, Bittner GD, Hubbell JA. Effects of fibrinolysis on neurite growth from dorsal root ganglia cultured in two- and threedimensional fibrin gels. The Journal of Comparative Neurology. 1996;**365**:380-391

[26] Boateng JS, Matthews KH, Stevens HN, et al. Wound healing dressings and drug delivery systems: A review. Journal of Pharmaceutical Sciences. 2008;**97**:2892-2923

[27] Sofia S, McCarthy MB, Gronowicz G, et al. Functionalized silkbased biomaterials for bone formation. Journal of Biomedical Materials Research. 2001;**54**:139-148

[28] Mota A, Sahebghadam Lotfi A, Barzin J, Hatam M, Adibi B, Khalaj Z, et al. Human bone marrow mesenchymal stem cell behaviors on PCL/gelatin nanofibrous scaffolds modified with a collagen IV-derived RGD-containing peptide. Cell Journal. 2014;**16**:1-10

[29] Rnjak-Kovacina J, Wise SG, Li Z, et al. Electrospun synthetic human elastin: Collagen composite scaffolds for dermal tissue engineering. Acta Biomaterialia. 2012;**8**:3714-3722

[30] Muzzarelli R. Human enzymatic activities related to the therapeutic administration of chitin derivatives. Cellular and Molecular Life Sciences. 1997;**53**:131-140

[31] Okamoto Y, Yano R, Miyatake K, et al. Effects of chitin and chitosan on blood coagulation. Carbohydrate Polymers. 2003;**53**:337-342

[32] Kweon D-K, Song S-B, Park Y-Y. Preparation of water-soluble chitosan/

heparin complex and its application as wound healing accelerator. Biomaterials. 2003;**24**:1595-1601

[33] Ueno H, Mori T, Fujinaga T. Topical formulations and wound healing applications of chitosan. Advanced Drug Delivery Reviews. 2001;**52**:105-115

[34] Fu L, Zhou P, Zhang S, Yang G. Evaluation of bacterial nanocellulose-based uniform wound dressing for large area skin transplantation. Materials Science and Engineering: C. 2013;**33**:2995-3000

[35] Dhandayuthapani B, Yoshida Y, Maekawa T, et al. Polymeric scaffolds in tissue engineering application: A review. The International Journal of Polymer Science. 2011;**2011**:290602

[36] Bhardwaj N, Sow WT, Devi D, et al. Silk fibroin–keratin based 3D scaffolds as a dermal substitute for skin tissue engineering. Integrative Biology. 2015;7:53-63

[37] Bragulla HH, Homberger DG. Structure and functions of keratin proteins in simple, stratified, keratinized and cornified epithelia. Journal of Anatomy. 2009;**214**:516-559

[38] Balakrishnan B, Mohanty M, Umashankar P, et al. Evaluation of an in situ forming hydrogel wound dressing based on oxidized alginate and gelatin. Biomaterials. 2005;**26**:6335-6342

[39] Chandika P, Ko S-C, Oh G-W, et al. Fish collagen/alginate/chito oligosaccharides integrated scaffold for skin tissue regeneration application. International Journal of Biological Macromolecules. 2015;**81**:504-513

[40] Gravante G, Delogu D, Giordan N, et al. The use of hyalomatrix PA in the treatment of deep partial-thickness burns. Journal of Burn Care & Research. 2007;**28**:269-274

[41] Cheng Y-L, Lee M-L. Development of dynamic masking rapid prototyping system for application in tissue engineering. Rapid Prototyping Journal. 2009;**15**:29-41

[42] Singh D, Singh MR. Development of antibiotic and debriding enzyme-loaded PLGA microspheres entrapped in PVA-gelatin hydrogel for complete wound management. Artificial Cells, Blood Substitutes, and Immobilization Biotechnology. 2012;**40**:345-353

[43] Amirthalingam M, Kasinathan N, Amuthan A, et al. Bioactive PLGA–Curcumin microparticle-embedded chitosan scaffold: In vitro and in vivo evaluation. Artificial Cells, Nanomedicine, and Biotechnology. 2017;**45**:233-241

[44] Cacciotti I, Ciocci M, Di Giovanni E, Nanni F, Melino S. Hydrogen sulfide-releasing fibrous membranes: Potential patches for stimulating human stem cells proliferation and viability under oxidative stress. International Journal of Molecular Sciences. 2018;**19**:2368

[45] Cacciotti I, Chronopoulou L, Palocci C, Amalfitano A, Cantiani M, Cordaro M, et al. Controlled release of 18-β-glycyrrhetic acid by nanodelivery systems increases cytotoxicity on oral carcinoma cell line. Nanotechnology. 2018;**29**:285101

[46] Kibe T, Koga T, Nishihara K, Fuchigami T, Yoshimura T, Taguchi T, et al. Examination of the early wound healing process under different wound dressing conditions. Oral Surgery, Oral Medicine, Oral Pathology, Oral Radiology. 2017;**123**:310-319

[47] Xie Z, Paras CB, Weng H, Punnakitikashem P, Su LC, Vu K, et al.

Dual growth factor releasing multi-functional nanofibers for wound healing. Acta Biomaterialia. 2013;**9**:9351-9359

[48] Lee S-H, Moon JJ, Miller JS, et al. Poly (ethylene glycol) hydrogels conjugated with a collagenase-sensitive fluorogenic substrate to visualize collagenase activity during three-dimensional cell migration. Biomaterials. 2007;**28**:3163-3170

[49] Keshel SH, Biazar E, Rezaei Tavirani M, et al. The healing effect of unrestricted somatic stem cells loaded in collagen-modified nanofibrous PHBV scaffold on full-thickness skin defects. Artificial Cells, Nanomedicine, and Biotechnology. 2014;**42**:210-216

[50] Zhou Y, Yang D, Nie J. Electrospinning of chitosan/poly (vinylalcohol)/acrylic acid aqueous solutions. Journal of Applied Polymer Science. 2006;**102**:5692-5697

[51] Bahrami H, Keshel SH, Chari AJ, et al. Human unrestricted somatic stem cells loaded in nanofibrous PCL scaffold and their healing effect on skin defects. Artificial Cells, Nanomedicine, and Biotechnology. 2016;**44**:1556-1560

[52] Hou J, Chen L, Liu Z, Li J, Yang J, Zhong A, et al. Sustained release of N-acetylcysteine by sandwich structured polycaprolactone/collagen scaffolds for wound healing. Journal of Biomedical Materials Research. Part A. 2019;**107**(7):1414-1424. DOI: 10.1002/jbm.a.36656. Epub 2019 Mar 5

[53] Chen G, Ushida T, Tateishi T. Scaffold design for tissue engineering. Macromolecular Bioscience. 2002;**2**:67-77

[54] Gunatillake P, Mayadunne R, Adhikari R. Recent developments in biodegradable synthetic polymers. Biotechnology Annual Review. 2006;**12**:301-347

[55] Place ES, George JH, Williams CK, et al. Synthetic polymer scaffolds for tissue engineering. Chemical Society Reviews. 2009;**38**:1139-1151

[56] Chen G, Ushida T, Tateishi T. Hybrid biomaterials for tissue engineering: A preparative method for PLA or PLGA–collagen hybrid sponges. Advanced Materials. 2000;**12**:455-457

[57] Shamis Y, Hewitt KJ, Bear SE, Alt-Holland A, Qari H, Margvelashvilli M, et al. iPSC-derived fibroblasts demonstrate augmented production and assembly of extracellular matrix proteins. In Vitro Cellular & Developmental Biology. Animal. 2012;**48**:112-122

[58] Singh H, Purohit SD, Bhaskar R, Yadav I, Bhushan S, Gupta MK, et al. Curcumin in decellularized goat small intestine submucosa for wound healing and skin tissue engineering. Journal of Biomedical Materials Research. Part B, Applied Biomaterials. 2022;**110**:210-219

[59] Zhang Q, Johnson JA, Dunne LW, Chen Y, Iyyanki T, Wu Y, et al. Decellularized skin/adipose tissue flap matrix for engineering vascularized composite soft tissue flaps. Acta Biomaterialia. 2016;**35**:166-184

[60] Wang B, Qinglai T, Yang Q, Li M, Zeng S, Yang X, et al. Functional acellular matrix for tissue repair. Materials Today Bio. 2023;**18**:100530

[61] Md Fadilah NI, M.S. MAKJ, Badrul Hisham MAI, Sunthar Raj N, Shamsuddin SA, Ng MH, et al. Cell secretomes for wound healing and tissue regeneration: Next generation acellular based tissue engineered products. Journal of Tissue Engineering. 2022;**13**:20417314221114273

[62] Chang DK, Louis MR, Gimenez A, Reece EM. The basics of Integra dermal

regeneration template and its expanding clinical applications. Seminars in Plastic Surgery. 2019;**33**:185-189

[63] Jansen LA, De Caigny P, Guay NA, Lineaweaver WC, Shokrollahi K. The evidence base for the acellular dermal matrix AlloDerm: A systematic review. Annals of Plastic Surgery. 2013;**70**(5):587-594. DOI: 10.1097/SAP.0b013e31827a2d23

[64] Mohd Hilmi AB, Halim AS. Vital roles of stem cells and biomaterials in skin tissue engineering. World Journal of Stem Cells. 2015;**7**:428-436

[65] Azari Z, Nazarnezhad S, Webster TJ, Hoseini SJ, Brouki Milan P, Baino F, et al. Stem cell-mediated angiogenesis in skin tissue engineering and wound healing. Wound Repair and Regeneration. 2022;**30**(4):421-435. DOI: 10.1111/wrr.13033. Epub 2022 Jun 14

[66] Takahashi K, Tanabe K, Ohnuki M, Narita M, Ichisaka T, Tomoda K, et al. Induction of pluripotent stem cells from adult human fibroblasts by defined factors. Cell. 2007;**131**:861-872

[67] Hu B-Y, Weick JP, Yu J, Ma L-X, Zhang X-Q, Thomson JA, et al. Neural differentiation of human induced pluripotent stem cells follows developmental principles but with variable potency. Proceedings of the National Academy of Sciences of the United States of America. 2010;**107**:4335-4340

[68] Villa-Diaz LG, Brown SE, Liu Y, Ross AM, Lahann J, Parent JM, et al. Derivation of mesenchymal stem cells from human induced pluripotent stem cells cultured on synthetic substrates. Stem Cells. 2012;**30**:1174-1181

[69] Zhang J, Guan J, Niu X, Hu G, Guo S, Li Q, et al. Exosomes released from human induced pluripotent stem cells-derived MSCs facilitate cutaneous wound healing by promoting collagen synthesis and angiogenesis. Journal of Translational Medicine. 2015;**13**:49

[70] Wong T, McGrath JA, Navsaria H. The role of fibroblasts in tissue engineering and regeneration. The British Journal of Dermatology. 2007;**156**:1149-1155

[71] Hassan WU, Greiser U, Wang W. Role of adipose-derived stem cells in wound healing. Wound Repair and Regeneration. 2014;**22**:313-325

[72] Li KN, Tumbar T. Hair follicle stem cells as a skin-organizing signaling center during adult homeostasis. The EMBO Journal. 2021;**40**:e107135

[73] Vu NB, Nguyen HT, Palumbo R, Pellicano R, Fagoonee S, Pham PV. Stem cell-derived exosomes for wound healing: Current status and promising directions. Minerva Medica. 2021;**112**:384-400

[74] Hart CE, Loewen-Rodriguez A, Lessem J. Dermagraft: Use in the treatment of chronic wounds. Advances in Wound Care (New Rochelle). 2012;**1**(3):138-141. DOI: 10.1089/wound.2011.0282

[75] https://www.epicel.com/treatment-with-epicel.html

[76] Zaulyanov L, Kirsner RS. A review of a bi-layered living cell treatment (Apligraf) in the treatment of venous leg ulcers and diabetic foot ulcers. Clinical Interventions in Aging. 2007;**2**:93-98

[77] Kim W-S, Park B-S, Sung J-H, Yang J-M, Park S-B, Kwak S-J, et al. Wound healing effect of adipose-derived stem cells: A critical role of secretory factors on human dermal fibroblasts. Journal of Dermatological Science. 2007;**48**:15-24

[78] Nourian Dehkordi A, Mirahmadi Babaheydari F, Chehelgerdi M, Raeisi Dehkordi S. Skin tissue engineering: Wound healing based on stem-cell-based therapeutic strategies. Stem Cell Research & Therapy. 2019;**10**:111

[79] Supp DM, Boyce ST. Engineered skin substitutes: Practices and potentials. Clinics in Dermatology. 2005;**23**:403-412

[80] Gungor-Ozkerim PS, Inci I, Zhang YS, Khademhosseini A, Dokmeci MR. Bioinks for 3D bioprinting: An overview. Biomaterials Science. 2018;**6**:915-946

[81] Singh D, Singh D, Han SS. 3D printing of scaffold for cells delivery: Advances in skin tissue engineering. Polymers. 2016;**8**:19

[82] Kim BS, Kwon YW, Kong JS, Park GT, Gao G, Han W, et al. 3D cell printing of in vitro stabilized skin model and in vivo pre-vascularized skin patch using tissue-specific extracellular matrix bioink: A step towards advanced skin tissue engineering. Biomaterials. 2018;**168**:38-53

[83] Wu Y, Liang T, Hu Y, Jiang S, Luo Y, Liu C, et al. 3D bioprinting of integral ADSCs-NO hydrogel scaffolds to promote severe burn wound healing. Regenerative Biomaterials. 2021;**8**(3):rbab014

[84] Nichol JW, Koshy ST, Bae H, Hwang CM, Yamanlar S, Khademhosseini A. Cell-laden microengineered gelatin methacrylate hydrogels. Biomaterials. 2010;**31**:5536-5544

[85] Xu L, Chen Y, Zhang P, Tang J, Xue Y, Luo H, et al. 3D printed heterogeneous hybrid hydrogel scaffolds for sequential tumor photothermal-chemotherapy and wound healing. Biomaterials Science. 2022;**10**(19):5648-5661

[86] Lin Z, Xie W, Cui Z, Huang J, Cao H, Li Y. 3D printed alginate/gelatin-based porous hydrogel scaffolds to improve diabetic wound healing. Giant. 2023;**16**:100185

[87] Duan H, Feng B, Guo X, Wang J, Zhao L, Zhou G, et al. Engineering of epidermis skin grafts using electrospun nanofibrous gelatin/polycaprolactone membranes. International Journal of Nanomedicine. 2013;**8**:2077-2084

[88] Pisani S, Dorati R, Chiesa E, Genta I, Modena T, Bruni G, et al. Release profile of gentamicin sulfate from polylactide-co-polycaprolactone electrospun nanofiber matrices. Pharmaceutics. 2019;**11**:161

[89] Thomas R, Soumya KR, Mathew J, Radhakrishnan EK. Electrospun Polycaprolactone membrane incorporated with biosynthesized silver nanoparticles as effective wound dressing material. Applied Biochemistry and Biotechnology. 2015;**176**:2213-2224

[90] Leu J-G, Chen S-A, Chen H-M, Wu W-M, Hung C-F, Yao Y-D, et al. The effects of gold nanoparticles in wound healing with antioxidant epigallocatechin gallate and α-lipoic acid. Nanomedicine: Nanotechnology, Biology and Medicine. 2012;**8**:767-775

[91] Yang X, Yang J, Wang L, Ran B, Jia Y, Zhang L, et al. Pharmaceutical intermediate-modified gold nanoparticles: Against multidrug-resistant bacteria and wound-healing application via an electrospun scaffold. ACS Nano. 2017;**11**:5737-5745

[92] Sabitha M, Rajiv S. Preparation and characterization of ampicillin-incorporated electrospun polyurethane scaffolds for wound healing and infection control. Polymer Engineering and Science. 2015;**55**(3):541-548

[93] Chen M, Przyborowski M, Berthiaume F. Stem cells for skin tissue engineering and wound healing. Critical Reviews in Biomedical Engineering. 2009;**37**:399-421

[94] Kanji S, Das H. Advances of stem cell therapeutics in cutaneous wound healing and regeneration. Mediators of Inflammation. 2017;**2017**:5217967

[95] Hussein SMI, Nagy K, Nagy A. Human induced pluripotent stem cells: The past, present, and future. Clinical Pharmacology and Therapeutics. 2011;**89**:741-745

[96] Yamanaka S. Induced pluripotent stem cells: Past, present, and future. Cell Stem Cell. 2012;**10**:678-684

[97] Nuschke A. Activity of mesenchymal stem cells in therapies for chronic skin wound healing. Organogenesis. 2014;**10**:29-37

[98] Ng WL, Wang S, Yeong WY, Naing MW. Skin bioprinting: Impending reality or fantasy? Trends in Biotechnology. 2016;**34**:689-699

[99] Tottoli EM, Dorati R, Genta I, Chiesa E, Pisani S, Conti B. Skin wound healing process and new emerging technologies for skin wound care and regeneration. Pharmaceutics. 2020;**12**(8):735. DOI: 10.3390/pharmaceutics12080735

[100] Sufiyan M, Kushwaha P, Ahmad M, Mandal P, Vishwakarma KK. Scaffold-mediated drug delivery for enhanced wound healing: A review. AAPS PharmSciTech. 2024;**25**(5):137. DOI: 10.1208/s12249-024-02855-1

[101] Jorgensen AM, Mahajan N, Atala A, Murphy SV. Advances in skin tissue engineering and regenerative medicine. Journal of Burn Care & Research. 2023;**44**:S33-S41

[102] Olson JL, Atala A, Yoo JJ. Tissue engineering: Current strategies and future directions. Chonnam Medical Journal. 2011;**47**:1-13